Praise for *Fighting Cancer from Within*

"*Fighting Cancer from Within* is an essential book for people with cancer. Dr. Rossman provides an impeccable guide to the use of imagery and other techniques in the cancer journey. He specifically addresses the different needs people with cancer have as they face diagnosis, treatment choices, surgery, chemotherapy, radiation, and other decisions. Speaking with wisdom, compassion, and clarity, Dr. Rossman has written a new classic to help people with cancer always to live better and, where possible, to live longer as well."

—Michael Lerner, president, *Commonweal*, author of
*Choices in Healing: Integrating the Best of Conventional
and Complementary Approaches to Cancer*

"*Fighting Cancer from Within* is illuminating, practical, and deeply reassuring. Dr. Rossman is a beautiful teacher and a wise healer."

—James S. Gordon, M.D., founder and director,
Center for Mind-Body Medicine, author of *Manifesto for
a New Medicine* and *Comprehensive Cancer Care*

"Dr. Rossman reminds us that we all possess the spirit and strength to regain control when cancer takes over our lives. His creativity and experience over the years are on full display in *Fighting Cancer from Within*, a bright and useful synthesis of imagery and other tools that can restore harmony and set the compass for smooth sailing in rough seas."

—Debu Tripathy, professor of medicine and director,
Komen Alliance Breast Cancer Research Center,
University of Texas Southwestern Medical Center

"For anyone determined to fight cancer and the side effects of cancer treatment, this book is mandatory reading. It will show you how to use guided imagery and the mind-body connection to stop worrying and to start winning to the very best of your ability."

—David E. Bresler, Ph.D, L.Ac., associate clinical professor of
anesthesiology, UCLA School of Medicine, codirector, Academy
for Guided Imagery, former White House commissioner on
Complementary and Alternative Medicine Policy

Also by Martin L. Rossman

Guided Imagery for Self-Healing

Fighting Cancer from Within

MARTIN L. ROSSMAN, M.D.

Fighting
Cancer
from
Within

❖

HOW TO USE
THE POWER OF
YOUR MIND
FOR HEALING

❖

An Owl Book
Henry Holt and Company   ✦   New York

To life

Owl Books
Henry Holt and Company, LLC
Publishers since 1866
175 Fifth Avenue
New York, New York 10010
www.henryholt.com

An Owl Book® and ® are registered trademarks
of Henry Holt and Company, LLC.

Library of Congress Cataloging-in-Publication Data
Rossman, Martin L.
   Fighting cancer from within : how to use the power
of your mind for healing / Martin L. Rossman.—1st ed.
      p.   cm.
   ISBN-13: 978-0-8050-6916-7
   ISBN-10: 0-8050-6916-X
   1. Cancer—Alternative treatment.   2. Cancer—
Psychosomatic aspects.   3. Stress management.   I. Title.
RC271.A62R677   2003
616.99'408—dc21   2002192217

Henry Holt books are available for special promotions
and premiums. For details contact: Director, Special Markets.

First Edition 2003

Designed by Victoria Hartman

Printed in the United States of America

3   5   7   9   10   8   6   4

Contents

Foreword

Adiagnosis of cancer is a personal encounter with the will to live, and this very useful and empowering book is about this will and how to befriend it in yourself.

The will to live is the impulse toward wholeness and integrity that is buried in the heart of every living thing. It is what enables us to meet illness and obstacles, survive them, and grow in spite them, and it is something one discovers not from reading a textbook, but from living a life. The will to live awakens in us any time that we are wounded, but most of us are unaware of the quickening of this power. Many people are living examples of the will to live and do not know it. Few of us trust the will to live in ourselves. Yet we who doubt are covered with the scars of many healings.

In my forty years of medical practice, people have often told me that they have recovered from their cancer because of chemotherapy, surgery, or radiation. They have come to feel so dependent on some form of treatment in order to survive that the end of treatment causes them uneasiness rather than celebration. Yet perhaps there is another way to think about this.

Cancer treatments may have the same effect on us that pruning has on a rosebush. These approaches create the conditions that give the will to live in us the best chance to express itself. Chemotherapy and radiation may be the means by which we recover but the reason that we recover may be something quite different, something we brought with us to our doctor's office and not something that we found there.

The will to live cannot be measured, which puts it beyond the reach of science. Science defines life in its own ways but life is larger than science. Many things happen that science cannot predict or explain. In the presence of cancer it is important to define life large. When we define life in ways that are too small we may define ourselves in ways that are too small as well.

These days, many people seem to hold themselves too small. Confronted by the daunting complexity of contemporary medicine they feel unable to participate and help themselves and can only surrender. When challenged with a life-threatening illness, it simply makes sense to use the full power of scientific medicine in your own behalf as well as drawing on the collective wisdom of the world's healing traditions. But each of us can also study the will to live in ourselves and befriend it. Developing tools to deliberately cultivate this power can help us not only to successfully meet with a diagnosis of cancer but can enable us, because of it, to learn to live more fully and passionately than ever before.

There are ways in which only we can help ourselves, ways that draw on our birthright as human beings. Imagination is a human power that is often overlooked in the search for healing. *Fighting Cancer from Within* will give you the tools to master your imagination and heal your life.

We each heal in ways that are as unique as our fingerprints. Dr. Rossman knows this, and in this book he takes us to the place of healing in us that is our own. With the sort of credibility that can only be gained through years of experience, he leads us step by step through the confusing stages and choices of the process of healing, offering us his expertise and his reassurance as we build our skills and find our strength. Anyone who needs to read this book will be blessed by it.

RACHEL NAOMI REMEN, M.D.
Author of *Kitchen Table Wisdom, My Grandfather's Blessings,*
Professor of Clinical Medicine,
University of California San Francisco, School of Medicine

Introduction

You can't know where life will take you,
but you can commit to a direction.
—*Wendell Berry*

If you have been diagnosed with cancer, and you want to have the best chance to survive it, then this book is for you. The way you use your mind can make a huge difference in what happens to you; the evidence points to effects that range from improving your emotional well-being to reducing adverse effects of treatments, to surviving, even thriving, through the experience.

This book will teach you techniques that can help you relax, reduce stress, relieve pain, and reduce adverse effects from treatments. It will also teach you methods that have been shown to stimulate immunity and other healing responses of the body, as well as methods for making difficult decisions and using your resources to best effect whether your goal is cure or comfort.

For the past thirty years I have helped people with cancer harness the power of their minds to fight their disease, find their strengths, make the best of treatments, and meet the challenges a significant illness brings. While many of the skills you will learn here have other uses in life, my focus will be using them to meet the challenges of cancer.

When you are diagnosed with cancer, you can find yourself overwhelmed with emotions at a time when you most need to keep your wits about you. I aim to teach you to reconnect with your own inner strengths and resources so you can make the best use of them when you most need them.

Cancer is many diseases, and the first thing most newly diagnosed people need to know is that having cancer does not mean they will die from it. More than 50 percent of cancers diagnosed today are curable through conventional medicine alone, and as many cancer patients get well as succumb to their illnesses. While you are alive you have hope, and you have options. You have will, imagination, and powerful natural healing abilities within you that you can stimulate by the use of your mind.

There are many ways to cope with or fight cancer, and this book will help you find the best ones for you. The major tools we will be working with are your attention, your intention, your will, and, most important, your imagination. I intend to help you learn ways of thinking that can tip the balance of health and illness in the direction of healing.

Cancer Care 101: Treating the Illness, Treating the Person

In cancer care there are two complementary goals of treatment. One, the usual medical goal, is to kill cancer cells and tumors, or reduce their numbers and their ability to grow, reproduce, and spread (metastasize). The other, perhaps best called the healing goal, is to support the well-being and resistance of the patient. Here I use *resistance* to stand for all the mechanisms, known and unknown, that protect us from the development and dissemination of cancer.

Conventional medical care for cancer has for many years concentrated on destroying tumors without paying much attention to supporting the patient as a whole person, with innate healing capacities. Until recently, most people put themselves in the hands of an oncologist (cancer specialist) and did what they were told. While you almost certainly need a good oncologist to prescribe and monitor your medical treatment, there is often much more to surviving cancer. Charles Smith, M.D., is a prominent urologist who specialized for years in treating men with prostate cancer, and then developed aggressive prostate cancer himself. After going through treatment, he wrote:

> Cancer is not just a lump in your body that can be cut out or killed by radiation or drugs. It alters every aspect of your life. Time and time again patients would tell me this. Some would even say that, in the end, it was the best thing that ever happened to them. Statements like this make no sense to a physician who is solely focused on the details of surgery, radiation therapy, or ablation. *I have come to the conclusion that you, as a patient, cannot simply allow the management of your cancer and your life to be limited by the narrow views of the physicians you encounter.*[1] (Emphasis Dr. Smith's)

Dr. Smith points to a major problem with the conventional approach to cancer. While it aggressively attempts to eliminate cancer cells, it does little or nothing to promote the health, vitality, and well-being of the person who is fighting that cancer. A poorly nourished, poorly supported person with cancer, overwhelmed by emotions, is likely to have a much more difficult time than one who is better nourished, better supported, and better balanced emotionally.

Years ago I moved into a new house with my wife and infant daughter. Next to the back windows around the baby's room there were a number of ailing bushes. Not being much of a gardener, I called one in. A leather-skinned fellow looking twice his actual age said that the bushes had four different infestations and needed to be sprayed with four different chemical pesticides. When I asked him if they were toxic, he lit up a cigarette and looked at me as if I was from Mars. "Nah," he said, drawing deeply on his smoke, "I've been using them for years and they haven't bothered me none."

Having a small child, I got a second opinion from an organic gardener, a pleasant young man who carefully examined the plants and their environment. He agreed completely with the diagnoses made by the first gardener, but his approach to treating them was quite different. He said, "These plants are pretty sick, but they haven't been well cared for in some time. Let's give them what they need and see what they can do on their own." He then showed me how to prune the deadwood, aerate the soil, fertilize the plants, and get them on a regular watering schedule. In four months the bushes had regained their health and thrown off the infections themselves. The next year, they even produced beautiful blossoms.

The difference between the approaches of these two gardeners is a perfect analogy for a strictly medical versus an integrated approach to cancer care. The plants may still have needed pesticides if they weren't able to recover themselves, but they would probably have needed smaller doses and fewer than the first gardener recommended. In the same way, you may well benefit from medical and surgical treatment, but you are likely to do much better with all therapies if your basic needs are attended to as well.

Supporting your innate healing abilities can only help you make the best use of any treatment you choose, and, alternatively, neglecting them is likely to make it more difficult for any treatment to work. As the second gardener said to me, "You know, if these plants don't get regular water and proper nutrients, all the pesticides in the world won't be able to cure them."

Supporting your health and eliminating your disease are two complementary approaches to healing that support and strengthen each other. In my experience, neither one works as well as both together.

You can use this analogy to see if there are any changes in your life that would support your own healing more effectively. Is there "deadwood" in your life—areas where you put energy that does not produce something of value to your well-being? Can you eliminate any of it? Are there pests and parasites that can be picked off? Are you giving yourself good nutrition and enough water on a regular basis? Is there an appropriate balance of light (joy) and shade (rest) for you? What could you do to make that balance more enjoyable for yourself?

Supporting your health makes it easier to tolerate treatments that can sometimes be difficult, and that in turn increases the likelihood that the treatments will work as desired. Methods of supporting your health and enhancing resistance to cancer generally fall into three categories: (1) nutritional support, ranging from improvement of diet to sophisticated individualized programs of nutritional supplementation with vitamins, minerals, herbs, essential fatty acids, and natural biological response modifiers; (2) mind-body approaches, ranging from support groups to counseling, to meditation, stress reduction, and guided imagery practices, and body-mind practices such as yoga, chi gung, tai chi, Jin Shin Jyutsu; and (3) systematic approaches with time-honored healing systems, such as traditional Chinese medicine or Ayurvedic medicine.

While the methods differ, their goal is the same—supporting and stimulating the vitality and function of the innate healing systems of the body, mind, and spirit. This idea is an ancient one, which perhaps we lost sight of in our enthusiasm for what modern medical treatment might be able to do. In traditional Chinese medicine this is known as *fu zheng* therapy. *Fu zheng* translates as "supporting the righteous." In China, *fu zheng* is not the sole therapy for cancer, but it is a useful complement to both traditional and modern means to eliminate tumors and cancer cells. Many studies have shown that good nutrition, herbs, acupuncture, and mind-body approaches are all effective in reducing adverse effects from conventional treatments, and very likely in improving treatment results.

This book will show you how to use guided imagery for this purpose. Guided imagery has become quickly and widely accepted as a useful adjunct in the treatment of people with cancer due largely to its ease of use, low cost, and rapid psychological benefits.[2] It has been shown to increase both the numbers and aggressiveness of natural killer cells when practiced over time,[3] has been shown to reduce complications from surgery,[4] relieve pain,[5] and reduce adverse effects of chemotherapy.[6] Imagery is a psychological and medical intervention likely to increase your odds of recovery.

The Inner Game of Cancer

In the spirit of improving health while reducing disease, you might say that this is not so much a book about treating cancer, but rather a book about treating yourself so that you can best mobilize the resources you have for fighting cancer. I call this the "inner game" of cancer—the use of attitudes, skills, and techniques that can help you get the most out of this experience, and tip the scales in your favor, especially if the game is close. Years ago, Timothy Gallway wrote bestselling books on the "inner games" of tennis and golf, encouraging players to relax and trust their innate abilities. The inner game of healing benefits from many of the principles that he described.

It may seem strange to think of healing as a game, and I mean no disrespect for the seriousness of the situation by my use of the term. Instead, I hope it helps you to realize that you can be a player in this game, that what you think and do has effects, if not on the cancer then certainly on you and those around you. The way you play this game can make a huge difference in your experience with cancer and your treatment, and it may well make a difference in whether or not you survive.

In many ways, beating cancer is an athletic performance, and all top athletes know the importance of the mental game. A common comment from professional athletes, whether football players, golfers, or race car drivers is "My goal is to put myself in a position to win." They know that if they are in condition, if they study the tendencies of their opponents, and if they focus and concentrate on what they want to accomplish, they will often be in a position to win. They also know that if they are well prepared, they will often perform at their peak and be more likely to win.

Along with knowing how to prepare themselves to do their best, athletes also know that sometimes things happen that are outside their control—a freak shot from half-court that goes in, or an opponent who scores 10 under par for the final round, or a bad call by an official. Sometimes you just get beat fair and square. No single game is a guaranteed victory, but if you keep putting yourself in position to win, you have the best chance of doing so, whatever your game, including fighting cancer.

Playing the mental game of cancer is very much like a performance or a competition. It demands focus, concentration, intention, a game plan, and a willingness to do your best. Having the best chance to win involves conditioning of the mind and body, and the time and energy commitment that goes with it. You may not like competition and prefer not to frame your life in the context of winning and losing. But I still think you can learn from this analogy by understanding that while you cannot always predict outcome, you can prepare yourself and aim for the best you can imagine, utilizing all your resources in the process.

How to Use This Book

This book is meant to help you face the challenges of cancer. You don't need to read it from cover to cover, but rather read it as it is most helpful to you. Go to the chapters and sections most relevant to you whenever you need them. Topics are clearly indicated in the chapter titles so you can find what you need when you need it.

The journey through cancer is not a linear process; it is often circular and repetitive, with decision-making, problem-solving, information-gathering, and life-affirming practices used over and over again. Consider this book a toolbox to help you build the kind of life you most desire throughout your treatment and recovery.

If I were teaching you to build a house, I'd first want to make sure you could measure things accurately, that you could cut wood with a saw, hammer nails, and drill holes. But then when you started building you wouldn't use these skills in rote sequence—first measuring the materials, then drilling the holes, cutting all the boards, and so on. Instead you'd use the different skills you have at appropriate times to build the different sections of the house.

The same is true when fighting cancer. If you are going to have surgery or chemotherapy, you may want to read the first three chapters then go directly to chapter 7, "Preparing for Successful Surgery" or chapter 8, "Making the Most of Chemotherapy." If you are gathering information, choosing practitioners, or making treatment decisions, work with those chapters first. Most people will find the first few chapters helpful as an introduction to the common challenges of cancer, the ways in which imagery can be helpful, and how to begin to apply it. After that, pick your chapters and sections depending on what is most important, most imminent, or of most interest to you. If you'd like to learn more about what imagery is and how it works, read chapter 4. Chapter 5 will teach you ways to amplify the effects of your healing imagery. Chapter 6 will explain a way to evaluate the information you gather, and teach you an imagery process to help you make treatment decisions once you have the information you need. Chapters 7 to 9 will teach you to use imagery to make the most of surgery, chemotherapy, radiation, or any other treatment you choose. Chapter 10 will teach you imagery techniques for relieving pain, and chapter 11 will address the transformational potential of a life-threatening illness. Chapter 12 addresses the welcome, yet tricky, challenges of adjusting to life after cancer.

I have tried to make this book as simple and accessible as possible without glossing over the complexities faced by people with cancer. To this end, every chapter has a brief summary at the end, a list of bulleted points that communicate the essentials about that chapter and the imagery processes it teaches. If you don't have the time or energy to read a lot, or if you already understand what the imagery is about and want to get to it quickly, review the chapter summary first, then go ahead and experiment with the imagery process in that chapter and see what you get from it. Spend some time afterward writing, drawing, and thinking about your experience. Create a Healing Journal for recording these and other important insights and thoughts you have as you go through the process. I'll give you some specific ideas about how to do that on pages 25 to 26.

If imagery is new to you, and you'd like to have more information before experimenting with it, read the entire chapter first, then use the script or tape of the script and work with it for a while. Always feel free to modify any imagery experience as is right for you—the purpose is to help *you* develop new skills that can support you as you deal with your diagnosis, treatment choices, treatments, and life decisions.

Whatever your approach, I strongly recommend that you explore Your Healing Place imagery script in chapter 1 and then the Meeting with Your Inner Healer imagery script in chapter 3. These two scripts will provide you with basic skills and resources you will be able to use in many ways. They will often be referred to in subsequent imagery processes.

For all the imagery explorations in this book, read through the script once before you immerse yourself in the imagery. Then decide whether you will record the script yourself, ask a friend to read it to you, or order the tapes or CDs I have professionally recorded. If you decide to record scripts yourself, use a calmly paced voice and leave pauses of about three to four seconds at the spaces marked by an ellipsis, three dots (. . .), so you can pay attention to your imagery as it develops. Leave about ten seconds where there are paragraph breaks. If someone else reads you the scripts, ask him or her to pause by lifting a finger or hand when you need more time to pay attention to the images that emerge.

I will warn you, however, that making your own tapes can be time-consuming and frustrating if you don't have good equipment, a sound-protected studio, and experience with the timing. I speak from experience, and though I don't want to discourage you from doing this, it may not be the best use of your time and energy right now. To make it easier for you I have studio-recorded all the scripts in this book. There is ordering information in the back of the book.

If you get stuck or confused when exploring the imagery processes you may benefit from working with a trained, experienced professional who can guide you as you learn to use imagery in your healing. The Academy for Guided Imagery has certified more than 750 health professionals in Interactive Guided Imagery[sm] who can help you with this. To find a qualified professional, visit our website at www.interactiveimagery.com or call 415–389-9325 and ask for a referral in your area.

Whichever way you choose to proceed, I encourage you to give yourself some time to experiment with each imagery process—and give yourself permission to be a beginner. Go through the imagery processes with an open-minded curiosity, exploring each one as a journey, and notice what happens for you. Take some time to write or draw any thoughts or associations that occur. If you've only reviewed the chapter summary you may want to read the supporting material after an exploration or two. It will deepen your understanding of the process.

Remember that there is no "right" experience to have, and look for what is most useful to you. Consider what you can learn from each process to help you move toward your desired goal, whether that goal is recovery, promoting healing responses, better coping, or cultivating comfort or peace.

May you be blessed, guided, and healed in your journey.

Summary

+ Cancer is frightening, but it is not a death sentence.
+ Comprehensive cancer care involves both destroying tumor cells and supporting the vitality and healing ability of the person.
+ The ways you use your mind can significantly help you in many ways in your journey with cancer.
+ This introduction contains important instructions for using this book most effectively as you move through your cancer treatment.

1

Cancer Diagnosis: Nightmare, Challenge, or Bump in the Road?

The diagnosis is cancer, but
what that means remains to be seen.
—*Rachel Naomi Remen, M.D.*

Almost everyone responds to the diagnosis of cancer with a period of shock, numbness, and disbelief. This is the mind's way of protecting us from having to process more information and emotion than we can handle, and it lasts for a variable period of time. As time passes, and you are able to better accept what's happening, the way you deal with this illness will depend on how you perceive it. The way you perceive it will likely be a product of how you generally react to a crisis, colored by your conscious and unconscious beliefs about cancer, its treatment, and its outcomes. The distress you will suffer early on will come more from this set of perceptions and beliefs than from the disease, and that is why it is important to address your reactions.

After the initial shock, people tend to have one of four common responses to their diagnosis: they perceive it as a nightmare, a challenge, a bump in the road, or they just stay numb throughout the whole experience and never really deal with it consciously. There are psychological benefits to each of these responses in the short run, but in the long run, there are advantages to adopting some attitudes over others. Fighting cancer is most often a marathon rather than a sprint, because modern cancer treatment has changed many cancer journeys from short-term illnesses to illnesses that people live with over long periods of time. Because one perspective may help you better than another, and because it is possible to change your perspective, your automatic response bears examination and questioning.

Assuming that your goal is survival, let's look at each of these responses to see what they may bring to your fight with cancer. Responding to a cancer diagnosis as a nightmare is probably the most common early response. Cancer has become a symbol in our culture for everything bad. Relentless, out of control, sneaky, evil, and deadly, it's the bogeyman of health. It brings up fear of pain, death, loss of control, surgeries and procedures, toxic chemotherapies, and damaging radiation. It may make you feel isolated, different than your peers, and even ashamed. It brings into your life something you don't want to have and something you can't ignore. It costs a great deal of time and money and affects the lives of everyone around you. It threatens to take your life. It's easy to see why you'd view it as a nightmare.

The first question I will encourage you to ask of your response is whether it serves you in your healing goals. Does this view help you if your goal is to overcome and survive this illness? Does it mobilize your will to fight? Your will to endure? Does it offer any hope, any bright spots, anything worth fighting for?

The one advantage I can see to the nightmare scenario is that it has the capability of mobilizing your anger and determination to overcome this intruder. I am reminded of an important bit of psychological insight that came my way courtesy of Mickey Mouse.

I was speaking at a conference on mind-body medicine held at the Disneyland Hotel several years ago. My friends and colleagues, two of the major researchers in mind-body effects on cancer, Drs. Carl Simonton and Jeanne Achterberg, were there, and we decided to go over to the theme park. As night fell, we worked our way over to the lagoon to see *Phantasmic*, having heard it was a great sound and light show.

The show was organized around Mickey Mouse, who appears onstage in his sorcerer's apprentice robes. He soon falls asleep and starts to dream, and at first his dreams, projected onto a fine mist sprayed over the lagoon, are of pleasant things from old Disney movies. But then his dreams start to go bad—dancing pink elephants start to become distorted and scary and characters from other movies start to appear—the Big Bad Wolf, witches, evil queens, and monsters of all kinds. The music becomes louder, cacophonous, disturbing, and the lighting casts a progressively ominous mood. At the climax of what now has become a full-fledged nightmare, the whole lagoon bursts into flames! It's a scene from Hades. A huge 30-foot dragon menaces Mickey onstage as the music comes to a crescendo pitch, and when the tension is at its highest and you don't know how he's going to survive, he suddenly pulls out his sword and says, in his high-pitched voice, "Hey, wait a minute! This is *my* dream!" and runs the dragon through. The flames disappear, the lights come on, the music becomes triumphant—Mickey is awake! He's taken control! The happy strains of "Zip-A-Dee-Do-Dah" ring over the lagoon as a Mississippi riverboat comes around the bend with all the Disney characters singing and dancing and waving with joy.

We were all astounded. Mickey Mouse had reminded us that things not only happen to us, but we happen to things as well. We can submit to our dragons or stand up to them and fight for ourselves if we choose. Carl Jung, the eminent Swiss psychologist, said that the challenge to the conscious mind when it faces the fears that can live in the unconscious is symbolized by the legend of St. George and the Dragon. His conclusion? "You may conquer the dragon or it may eat you, but one way or the other, you have to deal with the same dragon."

By focusing on the mind-body aspect of cancer, I'm not implying that cancer is a psychological disease. I am saying, however, that the psychology of how you respond to cancer can make quite a difference in both the quality and even the length of your journey with it. My concern about staying in the nightmare mode is that it is tiring, draining, and disempowering. It gives all the power to the disease. Seeing cancer as *only* a nightmare obscures any possibility of overcoming it or even learning anything valuable from the experience.

Dr. Julia Rowland, the director of the Office of Cancer Survivorship at the National Institutes of Health, reported a survey funded by the National Cancer Institute in which 2,000 women with breast cancer were asked the question, "Is there anything else about your experience as a breast cancer survivor that you would like to share here?" The reviewers were struck by the many reports of self-discovery, insight, hope, and resilience and commented that if you didn't know it was cancer that had prompted these discoveries you might well seek out what these women had experienced.

Nobody, including the patients who were the recipients of these unexpected benefits, would consciously choose to have cancer, but the point is that there are gifts that can come with cancer, and it seems that it would be a shame to go through it experiencing only the difficulties. Why not look for and cultivate any benefits, while simultaneously fighting the disease?

A second common response to cancer is to experience it as a "bump in the road." It is viewed as something that happens to some people, isn't particularly meaningful, there is treatment for it, and some people are cured and some are not. George is a seventy-year-old retired military man and a longtime smoker who finally quit a few years ago. When a spot was found on his lungs, he went through the process of diagnosis and treatment without any outward signs of distress, though I'm sure he was scared at times. He went through each step of the diagnostic and treatment process, trusting his doctor's recommendations, not seeking or needing a second opinion, not needing to know about alternatives, and simply accepting it as something that life brings, just as it had brought everything else he'd experienced.

He had a part of his lung removed, came through the surgery well, recovered, and was back playing golf a few months later. He doesn't talk about it, doesn't seem to worry about it, and doesn't seem to spend any time or energy on it. I've seen many other people take this route, and I admire and even envy people who meet life's challenges this way. But I'm not sure that this is a way of reacting that can be learned. I think it's a result of temperament, culture, and upbringing. If you're lucky enough to be a bump-in-the-roader you won't suffer the anguish of the nightmare responder or the excitement and even joy of the adventurer. Even so, you may find that a number of the imagery techniques offered in this book may be helpful in handling some of the stress you experience, preparing for treatments, and making difficult decisions.

A third common reaction is that some people respond to the diagnosis as a wake-up call, a challenge, or even an adventure. They may even seem relieved to let go of the day-to-day humdrum of life and be stimulated by a heroic challenge. Chuck was diagnosed with lung cancer in his early forties. The father of a young child, he was naturally shocked and scared, but soon settled into a typical (for him) attitude of "Okay, let's see what this brings and what we can make out of it." He learned everything he could about conventional and alternative treatments, and since conventional medicine really had little to offer him (unfortunately the tumor was not operable when it was discovered) he explored a great number of healers and healing methods, from nutrition to mind-body to traditional Hawaiian kahunas. He inspired many people with his attitude and optimism through even the most difficult parts of his journey and met each new challenge with courage and good humor. A good friend and astute observer remarked to me some time after Chuck's diagnosis, "You know, it's funny, but when Chuck was diagnosed with cancer, he seemed to relax!" It was true. Chuck was an adventurer at heart, and while he loved his family, friends, and his life dearly, maybe he wasn't cut out for a daily go-to-work life. He rose to the cancer challenge naturally and heroically, and it filled him with life and awareness. He fought hard to survive and met every turn in the road with both courage and curiosity.

There has been some scientific research about attitudes and outcomes in cancer which is worth looking at, although always with the caveat that your opportunity and challenge is to find the attitude that works the best for you. British researchers Watson, Greer, and associates looked at survival in women diagnosed with breast cancer.[1] They responded in four different ways: (1) Fighting Spirit—a desire to fight and conquer the disease; (2) Denial—no significant psychological response to diagnosis; (3) Resignation—acceptance of the situation, analogous to "bump in the road" response; and (4) Hopelessness and Helplessness—the nightmare response. When the research team looked at percentages of survival, the results reflected the same order as listed above, indicating that attitude and response is indeed linked to survival. Some other studies have not supported this finding, however. In 1998 Barrie Cassileth and others reviewed survival for people with advanced cancer three to eight years after their diagnosis. They were unable to link any psychosocial factor measured to length of survival.[2] It's important to realize that this is a very complex and difficult area to research. Outcomes vary depending on what you measure.

Here's some more encouraging data. The two studies mentioned above referred to people's initial adaptation or attitudes toward cancer and didn't look at what happens as people learn new coping skills or ways of dealing with the stresses and challenges that cancer can bring. A number of studies that do look at these factors are very encouraging.

One of the most powerful is a study by UCLA psychiatrist Fawzy Fawzy, M.D., of newly diagnosed patients with malignant melanoma. Fawzy compared randomized matched control subjects who had usual care with a group that participated in a six-week treatment soon after diagnosis.[3] This group, which met for only ninety minutes a week for six weeks, learned relaxation and active behavioral coping skills (ways to deal with stress), and had a chance to express their emotions and ask questions. Six years later Dr. Fawzy looked at the data and found that there was a remarkable advantage for the people who had been in the treatment groups. They were better adjusted, happier, and their immune system markers were much superior to control groups. Most important, in 34 patients in the treatment group there were only 3 deaths and 7 recurrences, compared to 10 deaths and 13 recurrences in the 34 patients in the usual care group.[4] Because of the randomized and prospective research design of this study, it is powerful evidence that people can learn to deal with cancer in ways that not only contribute to their well-being but to their chances of overcoming the cancer itself.

Another study by psychologist Dean Schrock investigating the effects of an eight-week group intervention for newly diagnosed breast and prostate cancer patients, based on the approach originated by Drs. Carl and Stephanie Simonton, showed similar results.[5] A more recent study by University of Toronto psychologist Alastair Cunningham looked at twenty-two people with medically untreatable metastatic cancer who participated in a weekly group for a year, learning relaxation, guided imagery, and other active coping and healing skills. Oncologists assessed the expected survival of the treatment group patients at the beginning of the year. After the year, the researchers classified the degree of involvement and participation with the skills taught and classified the participants into three categories—low, medium, and high levels of participation. They found that length of survival correlated well to the degree of participation in the group activities. They went further and looked at a number of psychological themes and found five especially correlated to survival. Cunningham states, "These themes were (1) the ability to act and change; (2) willingness to initiate change; (3) application to self-help work; (4) relationships with others; and (5) quality of experience. Results on a 5-point scale measuring the subject's expectancy that psychological efforts would affect the disease also showed a strong relationship to survival. In contrast, there was no relationship between survival and four standard psychometric measures taken at the onset of therapy.[6] It may be that using standard markers explains the Cassileth study's not identifying a correlation with survival.

Another perspective on attitudes and adjustment to, or survival from, cancer is emerging from studies conducted by psychologist John Astin at the California Pacific Medical Center in San Francisco. Astin refined Greer's model of fighting spirit versus resignation or hopelessness and found that women who could respond to challenges of breast cancer with both assertiveness *and* flexibility had the best adjustment and least distress, as compared to women who either rigidly attempted to maintain control or failed to try to assert control at all. In other words, in cancer, as with most things in life, there are times when responding with a fighting spirit is most helpful and there are times when acceptance is most helpful. The challenge is to discover which response is most appropriate at any given time. This, of course, is the subject of the well-known Serenity Prayer frequently used by 12-step groups: "Lord, grant me the courage to change the things I can change, the serenity to accept the things I cannot change, and the wisdom to know the difference." One of the effects I've noticed from the guided imagery techniques I'll teach you is that they often connect you to just those three things—courage, serenity, and wisdom—and help you to use each at the appropriate times.

So it's questionable that your *initial* response to a cancer diagnosis can predict your outcome, but there is much stronger evidence that *what you do next, and what you do over time has a greater influence—especially if you believe it can.* Whatever your initial response, you have the opportunity to learn new ways of using your mind, new ways of coping with stress, and new ways of supporting the innate healing systems of your body.

Whatever your usual way of dealing with difficulties, this book will teach you skills that can help you move from that initial reaction to one that can serve you better. To do that, you may well first need some help in order to manage what is usually the strongest and most common emotion to manage in dealing with cancer—fear.

Dealing with Fear

Dr. Larry LeShan, author of the book *Cancer as a Turning Point*, has said, "When you get diagnosed with cancer, every ghost and goblin of fear you have comes rushing though the rent that has been torn in the fabric of your self-identity." These fears are not only normal, they are almost inevitable, and we all handle them differently. Some people address fear head-on as a way of moving though it, while others avoid this because they are afraid that the fear might overwhelm them. You may try to ignore fear, or repress it, or get very busy so as not to have free time to dwell on it. Fear can be paralyzing if you let it, and though this may be a good time to be contemplative, it isn't a great time to enter a prolonged paralysis. There is great pressure from doctors, friends, and family, as well as from your own psyche to "do something" about this problem, and very little time to be with the emotions the problem is precipitating.

It's natural to have fears come up now, but it's also important to deal with your fears well. The high level of fear arousal you may feel at this time is somewhat useful in that it mobilizes you to find help and solve the problem, but if it is too strong and you can't break away from it, it can weaken you. You may experience high levels of anxiety, disturbed sleep, or loss of enjoyment, and depression may develop. But perhaps the most damaging thing about being overwhelmed by fear is that the fear may come between you and your strengths and resources, which are particularly needed at this time.

Emotions are inherently changeable. We're going to take advantage of that to help you learn some ways to shift your emotional experience when you want to or need to, and help you be more effective in your journey with cancer.

Following is a simple imagery experience to help you begin to shift how you feel. It will help you relax, begin to create a safe place of healing inside, and help you reconnect with your strengths. This is basically daydreaming on purpose—taking yourself in your mind to a beautiful, safe, and healing place, a place where you feel comfortable, cared for, and protected. This imagery relaxation process helps you to create a state of mental and physical relaxation in which your body's natural healing abilities can work without interference.

As with all the imagery processes you'll find in this book, let yourself explore and notice what happens as you go through it. Get comfortable in a place where you won't be interrupted for about twenty to thirty minutes. Let others know you need privacy during this time, and unless there's a true emergency, to avoid interrupting you. You could have

someone read the script below, in a calm voice, leaving a few seconds'
pause at the ellipses (. . .) for your imagery to develop and a little extra
time at the paragraph breaks. You can also record the script below yourself, then listen to it, or you can order my recordings of this and the
other imagery processes to guide you. However you decide to do it, let
it be an exploration and see how you imagine the things I suggest.

Your Healing Place

Take a comfortable position and let yourself begin to relax in your own
way . . . let your breathing get a little deeper and fuller . . . but
still comfortable . . . with every breath in, notice that you bring in
fresh air, fresh oxygen, fresh energy that fuels your body . . . and
with every breath out, imagine that you can release a bit of tension . . . a bit of discomfort . . . a bit of worry . . . and let that
deeper breathing and the thoughts you have of fresh energy in
and tension and worry out be an invitation to your body and mind
to begin to relax . . . to begin to shift gears . . . and let it be
an easy and natural movement . . . without having to force
anything . . . without having to make anything happen right
now . . . just letting it happen . . . just breathing and relaxing . . .
breathing and energizing. . . .

Come back to taking a few deeper breaths whenever you feel
like relaxing even more deeply . . . but for now, let your breathing
take its own natural rate and its own natural rhythm . . . and simply let the gentle movement of your body as it breathes allow you
to relax naturally and comfortably . . . almost without having
to try. . . .

And noticing how your right foot feels right now . . . and how
your left foot feels . . . and noticing that just before you probably
weren't aware of your feet at all . . . but now that you turn your

attention to them, you can notice them and how they feel . . . and notice the intelligence that is there in your feet . . . and notice what happens when you silently invite your feet to relax . . . and become soft and at ease . . . and in the same way noticing the intelligence in your legs and releasing your legs . . . and letting the intelligence in your legs respond in their own way . . . and noticing any release and relaxation that happens . . . without having to make any effort at all . . . just softening and releasing . . . and letting it be a comfortable and very pleasant experience. . . .

And you can relax even more deeply and comfortably if you want to . . . by continuing to notice the intelligence in different parts of your body and inviting them to soften and relax . . . and noticing how they relax . . . and you are in control of your relaxation and only relax as deeply as is comfortable for you . . . and if you ever need to return your awareness to the outer world you can do that by opening your eyes and looking around and coming fully alert . . . and if you need to respond to anything there you can do that . . . and knowing that you can do this if you need to . . . you can relax again and return your attention to the inner world of your imagination. . . .

Inviting the intelligence of your low back, pelvis, and hips to release and relax . . . and your abdomen and midsection . . . and your chest and rib cage . . . without effort or struggle . . . just letting go but staying aware as you do. . . .

Inviting the intelligence in your back and spine to soften and release . . . in your low back . . . mid-back . . . between and across your shoulder blades . . . and across your neck and shoulders . . . the intelligence in your arms . . . and elbows . . . and forearms . . . through your wrists and hands . . . and the palms of the hands . . . the fingers . . . and thumbs. . . .

Noticing the intelligence in your face and jaws and inviting them to relax . . . to become soft and at ease . . . and your scalp and forehead . . . and your eyes . . . even your tongue can be at ease. . . .

And as you relax, let your attention shift from your usual outer world to what we can call your inner world . . . the world inside that only you can see, hear, smell, and feel . . . the world where your memories, your dreams, your feelings, your plans all reside . . . a world that you can learn to connect with . . . that can help you in many ways on your journey. . . .

And imagine that you find inside a very special place . . . a very beautiful place where you feel comfortable and relaxed, yet very aware . . . this may be a place that you have actually visited at some time in your life . . . in the outer world or even in this inner world . . . or it may be a place that you've seen somewhere . . . or it may be a brand-new place that you haven't visited before . . . and none of that matters as long as it is a very beautiful place, a place that invites you and feels good to be in . . . a place that feels safe and healing for you. . . .

And let yourself take some time to explore this place . . . and notice what you imagine seeing there . . . all the things you see . . . and how you see them . . . don't worry at all about how you imagine this place as long as it is beautiful to you and feels safe and healing . . . and notice if there are any sounds you imagine hearing . . . or if it is simply very quiet in your healing place . . . notice if there is a fragrance or aroma that you imagine there or a special quality of the air . . . there may or may not be, and it's perfectly all right however you imagine this place of healing . . . it may change over time as you explore it, or it may stay the same . . . it doesn't matter at this point . . . just let yourself explore a little more. . . .

Can you tell what time of day it is? . . . or what time of year it is? . . . and what the temperature is like? . . . how you are dressed? . . . take some time to find a place where you feel safe

and let yourself get comfortable there . . . and just notice how it feels to imagine yourself there . . . and if your mind wanders from time to time, just take another deep breath or two and gently return your attention to this beautiful and healing place . . . just for now . . . without feeling the need to go anywhere else right now . . . or do anything else . . . just for now. . . .

And allow yourself to become aware of anything here that feels healing to you . . . it may be the beauty . . . it may be the sense of peacefulness . . . it may be the temperature, or the fragrance, or a combination of all the qualities that are here . . . perhaps you have a sense of what's sacred to you and what supports you in your life . . . it doesn't matter what you find healing here . . . or whether you can even identify it specifically . . . but let yourself experience whatever healing is there for you . . . and simply relax there . . . and know that while you relax, your body's natural healing systems can operate at their highest efficiency . . . without distraction . . . and without needing to be told what to do. . . .

The same built-in abilities to heal wounds, to repair injuries, to eradicate infections, and to destroy cancer cells that have been with you all your life can now function at full capacity . . . without any diversion of your precious energy . . . so while you relax, your body can take advantage of the time to fuel its ability to heal . . . as your muscles relax, your blood flows in all the right places . . . bringing your immune defenders to every place they are needed . . . and allowing them to efficiently and specifically target any cells that no longer belong to the healthy you . . . engulfing them and removing them . . . to be eliminated whenever you release what's no longer healthy for you . . . with your out breath . . . with your stool and urine . . . even with your sweat . . . and energizing yourself with fresh air and oxygen with every in breath . . . and with nutritious and healthy food . . . and with thoughts that bring you strength, courage, and even joy. . . .

And now let yourself become aware of the strength and power that you have within you . . . the strength that has seen you through all your life's other challenges . . . and the power of the energy that gave you life in the first place . . . that flows through you . . . and that sustains your life . . . and become aware of where you feel that most strongly in your body . . . and allow it to become even stronger if you like . . . a source of strength and power that you can draw from . . . and all you need to do is become aware of it and open yourself to feeling it. . . .

And as you welcome that feeling flowing through you, invite an image to form that represents that strength and power . . . and just let an image come to mind . . . take some time to observe the image that comes and notice how it represents and carries these qualitites of strength and courage . . . and perhaps a short phrase comes to mind that reminds you of this power . . . and whenever you want or need to reconnect with this strength and power, simply breathe deeply, relax, and think of this image and phrase . . . feel the strength within you and allow it to work for you . . . and let that be a good feeling. . . .

And taking all the time you need. . . .

(Pause for 30 seconds)

And now . . . when you are ready to return your attention to the outer world . . . silently express any appreciation you might have for having a special healing place within you . . . and for the healing capabilities that have been built into you by nature . . . and for feeling the strength and power you have within you . . . and for being able to use your imagination in this way . . . and when you are ready, allow all the images to fade and go back within . . . knowing that healing continues to happen within you at all times . . . and gently bring your attention back to the room around you and the current time and place . . . and bring back with you anything that seems important or interesting to bring back, including any feelings of comfort, relaxation, or healing . . . and when you are all the way back, gently stretch and open your eyes. . . .

And take a few minutes to write or draw about your experience.

Debriefing Your Experience

It's helpful to write or draw for a while after any imagery process. It helps you to recall and organize what you learn and experience, and makes the images available for review. As you periodically review your imagery and healing experiences, you will find that while they are imaginary, they also express an inner reality that is connected, coherent, and meaningful.

Take some time to write or draw whatever you noticed about your recent imagery experience. Don't worry about your artistic ability— this is just for you. Then write responses to the questions below and notice if answering them brings anything more to light.

How do you feel after doing this process?
Do you feel any different than you did before doing it?
What seemed important or interesting to you about this experience?
Do you feel you learned anything from this experience? If so, what?
What other thoughts or questions do you have about this experience?

Creating a Healing Journal

Although you can write or draw in any form about your imagery, I strongly recommend that you start a journal or diary of your healing experiences. You can call it your Healing Journal, or give it a title that's meaningful to you. Put anything in it that informs you, inspires you, or reminds you about healing—whether it comes from your imagery or from outside sources. Make it a sacred record that you can keep private or share with others, as feels right to you.

You can organize such a journal in many ways. You may want to make it chronological and record each day's insights, experiences, and feelings, or create sections for information about treatments, meaningful conversations, consultations, questions for your doctors and healers, questions for your inner healers, dreams that you relate to your healing journey, meditations, and, of course, your imagery. You can add quotations that move or inspire you to this journal, and photographs, articles, messages from friends, or anything that reminds you of your healing journey.

Create a journal that is attractive to you and that feels special and valuable. Conscious healing involves attention, concentration, dedication, and honesty. It's good to have a place to collect and express your innermost thoughts, feelings, insights, and questions, so make your Healing Journal an aesthetically special place in which to do this.

You may want to dedicate the journal in your own way, to consecrate it for yourself and define what goes in it. Reorganize it anytime you like—like your imagery and your life, it is uniquely yours.

Use the imagery process you have learned to relax, to go to your deep place of healing, and to build your strength until you feel ready to go on to the next imagery process. Reserve at least one or preferably two times a day when you will take about half an hour to practice your deep relaxation and healing imagery. Most studies that show the physiologic benefits of imagery cite a twice-a-day routine, although in a later chapter we'll customize that for you.

As you read on through this book, you will learn many other ways to use imagery to help yourself. The next chapter will focus on the tasks you face as a person newly diagnosed with cancer, help you identify your personal healing goals, and teach you another way to focus on your healing.

Summary

* Newly diagnosed people with cancer usually experience shock, numbness, and disbelief to some extent, and this is natural.
* After this, or accompanying this, comes a more personal reaction, generally based on how you handle a crisis or big change.
* Research indicates that there are skills and attitudes that are helpful for people with cancer, and that these skills can be learned and new attitudes considered.
* Managing fear and other strong emotions is often an important challenge in these early days and learning the guided imagery process in this chapter can help you with that.

2

After Diagnosis:
The First Three Weeks

I'm a strong believer that you should begin mind-body healing work as soon as possible after being diagnosed with cancer, assuming that healing is your goal. Although it's a difficult time, accompanied almost always by a sense of shock and disorientation, the sooner your mental resources are put into play the better.

Why? First, it may be weeks before you know what other kinds of treatments you can start, but you can start doing healing imagery no matter what type or stage of cancer you have. Imagery is something you can begin to do immediately that allows you to relax, moderate stress, and stimulate healing responses. Guided imagery practices return a sense of control—a sense that there is something you can do to help yourself while you go through diagnostic testing, wait for results, and educate yourself regarding treatment options.

Second, you are in a vulnerable emotional state. Studies show that after diagnosis nearly 60 percent of cancer patients are anxious or depressed, which is certainly understandable, but also usually treatable. Besides the suffering involved, anxiety and depression may also directly influence your survival because of the effects on your decisions and ability to follow through with treatment plans. More than 30 percent of chemotherapy patients prematurely quit treatment because of their emotional difficulties.[1] Immune functions can also be negatively affected by anxiety and depression, or by the effects anxiety and depression have on self-care, and you need your immune defense systems to be as functional as possible. Drug therapy for anxiety and depression is often helpful, at least in the short run, but we don't know enough about the effect these drugs have on cancer. There is some disturbing evidence that at least one drug therapy for depression can affect cancer recurrence. In a study published in the *Journal of Epidemiology* in May 1999, women with breast cancer who took the antidepressant Paxil had seven times the recurrence rate of women who took other antidepressants. While this finding has not been replicated and may be a red herring, it makes sense to choose another drug if you need an antidepressant. Imagine if the study had shown that ginseng or vitamin C was associated with this result—every doctor in America would be warning their patients not to use those substances—and with good reason. So if you can get a handle on your emotions without drugs you are better off. If you can't, medications can help you get back in control, and once you're back in control, you can see if you can discontinue them with the help of your prescribing doctor.

The third good reason to begin mind-body practices early is that your mental and emotional state may be important not only to you but to your family and close friends. Your family and friends might want to learn some relaxation and imagery techniques along with you, both to help themselves manage their stress and to support you better.

A fourth reason to begin mind-body interventions right away is that you may decide to begin chemotherapy, radiation, or surgery treatments fairly early in your journey. Although these treatments are often helpful, they can be accompanied by varying degrees of fatigue that interfere with the ability to concentrate or think clearly. "Chemo brain" is a common after-effect of many chemotherapy drugs, and radiation, surgical anesthesia, and postoperative medications may cause varying levels of fatigue and trouble with concentration and memory. A few weeks or even days of concentrated practice with imagery before you go through such treatments will help you to familiarize yourself with the practices and get you off to a good start. Besides, the healing imagery processes can help you minimize problems and increase the likelihood that the treatments will be helpful to you.

Tasks of the First Three Weeks

The tasks of this stage are threefold: (1) managing your emotional reactions without getting buried under them or collapsing; (2) gathering the information you need about treatment options, doctors, and other support resources; and (3) making the best decisions for you. This may be a cycle you will repeat more than once as you go through cancer treatment since not all successful treatment takes place in one shot. You may choose multiple therapies and sometimes there may be recurrences and the need for further treatment. If so, you may cycle through these stages again.

In the weeks after your diagnosis you will be bombarded with more information than you ever wanted to know about cancer and the options available for treatment. You will meet more doctors during this time than you may have ever visited in your life, and they may or may not agree about your optimal course of treatment. If you are alternatively minded, or simply want to augment your treatment by building your vitality in other ways, you may also be interviewing a host of complementary and alternative practitioners whose orientations are likely to vary even more than your physician's. You may well have a stack of books, videos, and audiotapes from well-wishers that you couldn't go through in half a year if you wanted to, and you will probably be contacted by lots of people with information, offers of help, questions about your condition, and stories about cancer. There will likely be a mixture of people who genuinely care for you and could be helpful, along with people who need to assuage their own fears, people who need something from you, people who need to convince you about their personal views of healing, and people who are simply nosy.

While going through this uninvited process you are likely to be disoriented, frightened, and in a state of disbelief. The whole progression of events may seem surreal, as if it is all happening to someone else, and events may seem to be unfolding without your participation or permission. This is quite normal and almost to be expected.

I will address ways of dealing with all these phenomena, but first you must clarify your personal goals for this period. Since you've never dealt with this situation before, you aren't likely to know what your goals are, but for most people they are simple (if not easy), and I would encourage you to keep them simple. This is a stressful and unusual time for you, and you need to focus on the tasks that are really most important to you. You've already begun to learn how to reduce your fear and stimulate your healing responses with the Healing Place imagery you learned in chapter 1, and we'll examine information gathering and decision making in more detail in chapter 6.

Clarify Your Goals

It's very helpful to write down your personal goals for the long term and for these first three weeks. This will help you see that this is the beginning of a process that will unfold over time and that there are choices you can make that will make a difference. You will go through different phases in your battle with cancer, and each phase will require different strategies, depending on your goals.

To clarify your long-term goals with your healing, prioritize them, and write them down in your journal. Having these goals in writing will help you make many decisions as you go along.

One woman I worked with found that placing "eradication of cancer from my body" as her number one overall goal was helpful to her in deciding how to spend her time and energy as she went through treatment. As she reviewed her goals every day, she found her awareness of this primary goal influenced the way she ate, the amount of exercise and rest she got, and her ability to say no to things that she felt didn't support this objective. She said she got to the place where every choice she made could either support her healing or work against it and used that as her benchmark. Another patient found that his goal of "Healing my mind, body, and spirit" allowed him to be more aware of how important the people around him and his meditation practice was to his well-being. It made him realize that his chemotherapy was an important part of his treatment for cancer, but that there was much more he could do to participate. Having this awareness allowed him to go through his treatment feeling much more of a whole person.

Take whatever time you need to write down your goals and objectives for your experience with cancer. This is for you. No goal is objectively better than another, so be true to yourself. Make your goals genuinely important to you. What is your number one goal for this experience with cancer? Your second most important goal? Your third? Also write down any other goals you have for this time.

After you've written them down, ask yourself each of the following questions in relation to each of your long-term goals, and write your answers in your Healing Journal.

What outer resources (people, information, things) do I need in order to accomplish this goal?

What inner resources (skills, qualities, strengths) do I need in order to accomplish this goal?

Where can I get the resources I need?

What might stand in the way of accomplishing this goal?

How will I deal with these barriers should they occur?

Now that you have clarified your overall objectives, get clear on your goals for the next three weeks. Try to be realistic and realize that you can only do so much in this short time. If you have more than five goals for this time be sure to prioritize them in order of importance to you, so if you need more time the most important ones will be handled first. Make sure to clarify your number one goal, and then your top three goals, so you can concentrate on them if you find there's not enough time to get further down your list. There will likely be time for other goals later. Record in your Healing Journal:

What is my number one goal for these three weeks?
What is my second most important goal for these three weeks?
What is my number three goal for these three weeks?
What other goals do I have for this time?

Once you've identified these goals, answer the same questions you did with your long–term goals.

Become a Worry Warrior

I sometimes joke that the most common form of imagery is called worrying. When you worry, you are repeatedly going over fearful and troublesome thoughts in your mind. Worries cause stress reactions and fear in your body through the same mind-body connections that mediate the positive effects of healing thoughts and imagery. Thus if you find yourself worrying a great deal during this time (like most people), it's helpful to know how to reverse that process and use it for healing instead.

Before learning to do that, however, realize that worry has a function. Worry lets you examine a situation from many angles as you look for a solution. It's like the process of untangling the knots in a big ball of string—you keep turning it over and over looking for places to loosen it and free up more string. The natural fears and concerns one has in this early stage of fighting cancer naturally leads to worry in most people. There's a point, though, where worry stops being useful and becomes simply stressful, interfering with your ability to rest, sleep, or concentrate on other issues that may be important.

In chapter 1 you learned an imagery process that can help you relax, begin to imagine healing, and feel stronger. This second imagery process will help you identify an image and perhaps a phrase that can symbolize your healing intention and teach you how to use them to replace futile worry.

The Worry Warrior imagery is a great antidote, because whenever you find yourself worrying, and whenever you decide to stop it, you can replace your worrying thoughts with an image and affirmation of the healing process as you intend and imagine it. Once you learn this process, the more you tend to worry, the more you will end up doing healing imagery.

Chapter 5 will teach you in detail a variety of different ways to augment your healing and recovery imagery, but for this process, I'll keep it simple and straightforward. Once you are relaxed, in an imaginary place that is healing to you, you'll be invited to create an image of your healing and an affirmation to accompany it. This image will act as a counter-response to your tendency to worry, and help you develop a "positive worry" habit.

Here's how it works: say you create an image of your healing process, or of yourself healthy and enjoying your life a few years down the road, or maybe an affirmation statement like "My body is a lean, mean self-healing machine." You then find yourself worrying about the cancer getting the best of you. You take a minute to consider whether this worry is about something you can act on; for example, if you find yourself worrying about making sure your insurance papers are in a place where your family can access them, it's something real that you can take care of, whether you do it yourself or delegate it. But if it's simply diffuse worry or anxiety, it's not helping you and may drain energy you can better use for healing.

When you've learned to be a Worry Warrior you will take a deep breath or two, relax, and imagine that you have a rubber stamp with a big red circle with a slash through it to cancel your thought/worry and then slide in your affirmation or positive image in its place. In a sense, you're saying to yourself (and you may want to actually say this to yourself), "This is my fear—it's real, but it's only a fear. Instead, here's what I want to have happen. Here's what will happen if it's up to me. I choose to energize and affirm my healing now." Take a lesson from Mickey Mouse: acknowledge your fears but don't let them push you around.

Following is an imagery script that will help you form a trigger image of healing and an affirmation. As always with these processes, let yourself explore and notice what happens as you go through it. You can repeat it as often as you like in order to refine or develop your images and affirmations.

Find a comfortable place where you won't be interrupted for about twenty to thirty minutes. Let others know you need privacy during this time and to avoid interrupting you unless there's a true emergency. Have your Healing Journal and drawing materials close at hand. Read through the script once so you'll know what's coming, and, if you don't have the prerecorded tape or CD, decide whether you will ask someone to read it to you or record the script yourself. However you decide to do this, let it be an exploration.

Worry Warrior Imagery

Take a comfortable position and let yourself begin to relax in your own way . . . let your breathing get a little deeper and fuller . . . but still comfortable . . . with every breath in, notice that you bring in fresh air, fresh oxygen, fresh energy that fuels your body . . . and with every breath out, imagine that you can release a bit of tension . . . a bit of discomfort . . . a bit of worry . . . and let that deeper breathing and the thoughts you have of fresh energy in and tension and worry out be an invitation to your body and mind to begin to relax . . . to begin to shift gears . . . and let it be an easy and natural movement . . . without having to force anything . . . without having to make anything happen right

now . . . just letting it happen . . . just breathing and relaxing . . . breathing and energizing. . . .

Come back to taking a few deeper breaths whenever you feel like relaxing even more deeply . . . but for now, let your breathing take its own natural rate and its own natural rhythm . . . and simply let the gentle movement of your body as it breathes allow you to relax naturally and comfortably . . . almost without having to try. . . .

And noticing how your right foot feels right now . . . and how your left foot feels . . . and noticing that just before you probably weren't aware of your feet at all . . . but now that you turn your attention to them, you can notice them and how they feel . . . and notice the intelligence that is there in your feet . . . and notice what happens when you silently invite your feet to relax . . . and become soft and at ease . . . and in the same way noticing the intelligence in your legs and releasing your legs . . . and letting the intelligence in your legs respond in their own way . . . and noticing any release and relaxation that happens . . . without having to make any effort at all . . . just softening and releasing . . . and letting it be a comfortable and very pleasant experience. . . .

And you can relax even more deeply and comfortably if you want to . . . by continuing to notice the intelligence in different parts of your body and inviting them to soften and relax . . . and noticing how they relax . . . and you are in control of your relaxation and only relax as deeply as is comfortable for you . . . and if you ever need to return your awareness to the outer world you can do that by opening your eyes and looking around and coming fully alert . . . and if you need to respond to anything there you can do that . . . and knowing that you can do this if you need to . . . you can relax again and return your attention to the inner world of your imagination. . . .

Inviting the intelligence of your low back, pelvis, and hips to release and relax . . . and your abdomen and midsection . . . and your chest and rib cage . . . without effort or struggle . . . just letting go but staying aware as you do. . . .

Inviting the intelligence in your back and spine to soften and release . . . in your low back . . . mid-back . . . between and across your shoulder blades . . . and across your neck and shoulders . . . the intelligence in your arms . . . and elbows . . . and forearms . . . through your wrists and hands . . . and the palms of the hands . . . the fingers . . . and thumbs. . . .

Noticing the intelligence in your face and jaws and inviting them to relax . . . to become soft and at ease . . . and your scalp and forehead . . . and your eyes . . . even your tongue can be at ease. . . .

And as you relax, let your attention shift from your usual outer world to what we can call your inner world . . . the world inside that only you can see, hear, smell, and feel . . . the world where your memories, your dreams, your feelings, your plans all reside . . . a world that you can learn to connect with . . . that can help you in many ways on your journey. . . .

And imagine that you find inside a very special place . . . a very beautiful place where you feel comfortable and relaxed, yet very aware . . . this may be a place that you have actually visited at some time in your life . . . in the outer world or even in this inner world . . . or it may be a place that you've seen somewhere . . . or it may be a brand-new place that you haven't visited before . . . and none of that matters as long as it is a very beautiful place, a place that invites you and feels good to be in . . . a place that feels safe and healing for you. . . .

And let yourself take some time to explore this place . . . and notice what you imagine seeing there . . . all the things you see . . . and how you see them . . . don't worry at all about how you imagine this place as long as it is beautiful to you and feels safe and healing . . . and notice if there are any sounds you imagine hearing . . . or if it is simply very quiet in your healing place . . . notice if there is a fragrance or aroma that you imagine there or a special quality of the air . . . there may or may not be, and it's perfectly all right however you imagine this place of healing . . . it may change over time as you explore it, or it may stay the same . . . it doesn't matter at this point . . . just let yourself explore a little more. . . .

Can you tell what time of day it is? . . . or what time of year it is? . . . and what the temperature is like? . . . how are you dressed? . . . take some time to find a place where you feel safe and let yourself get comfortable there . . . and just notice how it feels to imagine yourself there . . . and if your mind wanders from time to time, just take another deep breath or two and gently return your attention to this beautiful and healing place . . . just for now . . . without feeling the need to go anywhere else right now . . . or do anything else . . . just for now. . . .

And as you relax in this special place of healing, let an image come to mind that can symbolize the healing that is already going on within you . . . and the strength and abilities of the healing systems built into your body . . . simply allow an image to come that represents this to you—it may come in any form—perhaps it looks like you, radiant with energy or light . . . perhaps you can imagine and even feel the surging response of your immune defense system mobilizing to rid your body of any cells that have lost their way and need to be destroyed . . . perhaps it's an image of you in the future, healthy and well . . . but it could be anything . . . how would you imagine yourself full of healing energy and vitality and feeling whole, healthy, and strong? . . . let yourself begin to imagine yourself that way now . . . and don't worry at all about whether the image you have now is the best image or the strongest image . . . you may be aware of many images of your healing as you work through this process . . . and you may change your imagery many times to better fit your understanding of the process . . . but for now, let an image stabilize . . . and let this image be a symbol for the healing your body, mind, and spirit can do . . . and imagine it happening now in you . . . and imagine it being as strong and powerful and effective as you possibly can . . . if you need more power, imagine you can connect to people and things you love . . . and to whatever source of life and energy you imagine put you here in the first place . . . and imagine that those provide powerful sources of healing energy that you can direct throughout your body, mind, and spirit to heal what needs to be healed . . . to eliminate what needs to be eliminated . . . and to repair what needs to be repaired. . . .

Take a few minutes now and imagine this happening in your own way and let whatever way you imagine this happening to be just fine for now . . . your unconscious mind understands what your conscious mind is telling it . . . it understands that your intention is to activate and stimulate all the healing capabilities it has . . . and it knows just how to respond, however you imagine this healing. . . .

Let this be your image of healing for now . . . let a particular image or "film clip" of imagery come to stand for this whole process . . . and let a word or phrase come to mind that also represents this healing process . . . a word or phrase that both represents and stimulates this feeling of healing within you . . . it may be something you've heard, or something that just comes to mind right now. . . .

Give yourself time to settle for now on a word or phrase that can remind you of this healing that is happening and that you intend. . . .

(Pause for 20 seconds)

And now let your thumbs touch another of your fingertips and let that movement also symbolize and connect you with the feelings and process of healing within you . . . and anytime you make that subtle movement in the future, it can instantly reconnect you to the feelings of this healing process within you, and your image and phrase that further reminds you of the healing ability you have. . . .

And so anytime in the future that you find yourself worrying about cancer or how it will affect you, let yourself consider whether it serves you to think about that . . . and if it does, let yourself think creatively about how you can resolve that concern or further contribute to your body's ability to heal . . . but as soon as you become aware that your fears and worries are simply fears or worries, simply acknowledge them . . . and take a deep breath to begin to relax . . . and imagine that you cancel the fear or worry . . . you can imagine having a big red circle stamp with a slash through it and stamp that worry out . . . and touch your thumbs to those fingers . . . and become aware of your image of healing . . . and the word or phrase that reminds you of your intent to heal . . . and let that symbol and imagery of healing fill your awareness . . . and notice how it feels to imagine that healing happening in you now . . . imagining that you can feel it in your body . . . and knowing that the more you tune into this, the easier it is to imagine and feel . . . and that the more you do this, the stronger your ability to support your healing becomes. . . .

And you can let any good feelings that come with imagining healing this way grow stronger within you . . . and stay with you as long as you like . . . and even bring them back with you when you decide to return your attention to the outer world . . . knowing that healing is always happening within you . . . and the more you encourage it the stronger it can become. . . .

And taking all the time you need . . . and when you are ready to return your attention to the outer world, silently express any appreciation you might have for having a special healing place within you . . . and for being able to use your imagination in this way . . . and for the healing capabilities that have been built into you by nature . . . and when you are ready, allow all the images to fade and go back within . . . knowing that healing continues to happen within you at all times . . . and gently bring your attention back to the room around you and the current time and place . . . and bring back with you anything that seems important or interesting to bring back, including any feelings of comfort, relaxation, or healing . . . and when you are all the way back, gently stretch and open your eyes. . . .

And take a few minutes to write or draw about your experience.

Debriefing Your Experience

Take some time to write and draw in your Healing Journal about this experience. Some suggestions:

+ A drawing of your image/symbol of healing
+ A word or phrase that affirms this healing intention
+ The movement to make to reconnect to this experience
+ How you imagined healing happening in you
+ How it felt to do this
+ What seemed important or interesting about this experience
+ What you learned from this experience
+ How you will use it in the future

What's most useful about this Worry Warrior technique is that the more prone you are to worry, the more you end up doing healing imagery. Eventually it will become a habit and you'll have converted the power of your fear to the power of your will and imagination. It works. Try it—and stick with it. Experiment with it, simply touching your thumbs to those fingers, and recalling the healing images and words whenever you like or need to throughout the day. You might take three deep breaths and focus on them for a minute . . . or simply become aware of them in your mind as you are doing other things. Find the ways that work best for you. If you're really a good worrier, you may have to do this thought switching hundreds of times a day at first, but just patiently keep doing it whenever you become aware that your fears are up and you'll get to be a good Worry Warrior pretty quickly.

At this point, think about how you're doing with the goals you identified in this chapter. If you're still feeling that managing and reducing your stress is priority number one, proceed to the next chapter to learn some other ways to work with your feelings and reduce your stress.

Whichever chapter you choose to read next, set aside at least one, and preferably two or more times in the day to relax and work with your healing imagery. Do the processes that are most relevant to you as you learn them. Regular practice will make your imagery more effective, help to keep your stress level down, and help you do whatever else you need to do more effectively.

Summary

- The first few weeks after a cancer diagnosis are a time of disorientation, emotional shock, and pressure to find the best treatment.
- Clarify and prioritize your long-term overall goals in regard to your cancer and treatment. Once you do this, identify and prioritize your goals for the first three weeks. Goal setting helps you organize your priorities and helps you see that this is a process—and that you can't do everything at once.

◆ For most people with cancer, the most pressing immediate goals are to manage the strong emotions and stress; to gather information to help you navigate the medical options; and make initial treatment decisions.

◆ Learning the Worry Warrior imagery process in this chapter will help you convert worry to a positive habit and help you feel more in control of yourself.

◆ From here, choose the chapters you read by what is most important to you at this time.

3

❖

Combating the Stress of Cancer

Stress and emotional turmoil cause the majority of any suffering in the weeks after being diagnosed with cancer. Jeff Kane, M.D., author of *The Healing Companion* and a leader of cancer support groups for twenty years, says, "In the early days the tumor itself is usually very small—the devastation we can feel comes from its effects on our self-image, and the liberation of our worst fears. You get diagnosed and it's like you've been kidnapped and taken to a foreign country. You don't know anyone there and it's lonely and scary. Almost any contact can help and a skillful guide can be invaluable."

This chapter will teach you imagery techniques that will connect you to internal sources of support—your own ability to create peacefulness and strength—and help you access the wisdom within you. But first, let's discuss finding and using external sources of support, which is often crucial, especially in the early weeks and months following diagnosis.

Because so many tasks need to be completed during this time, and because there is so much variability of opinion about how to treat many cancers, finding someone you can rely on as a navigator or guide is very important. Usually this will be a physician, either your primary care doctor or an oncologist, a doctor that specializes in treating cancer. If you are considering alternative treatments (rather than complementary[1]) I still would recommend that you visit an oncologist or two to find out what conventional medicine has to offer you. You can always decline the offer.

Ideally, you will find a physician or other professional with special knowledge about cancer, one in whom you have confidence and whom you feel you can talk to and understand. There should be a feeling of mutual respect between you and this person and a sense that your goals and philosophy about treatment are well aligned. If your philosophy of medicine and healing isn't well aligned with your conventional physician, you may need to find a holistic or integrative physician, a nurse, a consultant, or even the new breed of health paraprofessional, the cancer guide or navigator, who has special training in helping people sort through cancer's complex weave of sometimes conflicting information. The Center for Mind Body Medicine in Washington, D.C., under the leadership of James Gordon, M.D., trains cancer guides and may be able to help you find one. Contact information can be found in Resources.

While you are the world expert on you, almost everyone needs to find a doctor or other cancer professional they feel they can trust. You are the one who knows (or at least has the best chance of knowing) your goals, what you are willing to tolerate, and what approach to healing makes the most sense to you. Ideally, you will find a doctor who respects that and can honestly communicate how they can help, and you will be able to work together toward the goals you set.

A recent *New York Times* article likened the choice of your physician, or whoever you pick as the leader of your cancer treatment team, to a pioneer family choosing a wagonmaster to lead them to the far lands of Oregon or California in the 1800s. They knew they were facing a long trip fraught with perils that they hoped would take them to a "promised land." Drought, heat, hostile Indians, epidemic disease, getting lost, prairie storms and flash floods were all likely, and if they set out too late in the year they ran the risk of getting caught in the mountain passes and freezing to death. A significant number of pioneers setting out in those days did not make it, and many of those who did suffered the loss of at least one important family or community member. Yet they did set out, with the possibility of a better life drawing them through their journey.

The pioneers had to make many important decisions about the supplies, equipment, and route they would take. Perhaps the most important was choosing the wagonmaster, the man who would lead them through this dangerous and unforgiving terrain. The decision you make about who to work with to treat you and your cancer is similarly important. What would you ideally want in a wagonmaster?

You certainly want someone with experience in treating people with your kind of cancer. You wouldn't want a wagonmaster who'd never made the trip before. Just as you'll want an experienced oncologist. An oncologist should also be a person of sound judgment, who can respect your values even if he or she doesn't necessarily share them. You want a doctor who is thoughtful, sensitive to the psychological and emotional trials of cancer therapy, and someone who cares. It's not only nice to feel cared for, but it lets you know that your doctor will do his or her best for you.

Many wagonmasters in the Old West were authoritarian. The rule was you did what they said. They knew the way and you didn't. They were the guides and that was their job. They had both a need and a right to be protected from unnecessary danger in the course of the trip. They didn't feel they had the time or desire to argue with people who knew little or nothing about the trip. Some doctors feel the same way, and if you trust them, that's fine.

Don't forget that a physician, whether an oncologist or not, may be put at serious risk by being asked to venture into unfamiliar territory in your healing path. Physicians are judged by the standards of practice in their community. If you want a doctor to treat your cancer with European mistletoe extracts and thymic hormones, it might sound like starting out on the Oregon Trail and getting a request (or demand) for a side trip through hostile territory on your way. Such a trip might dangerously delay your journey, or expose you (and him) to unknown dangers. So keep all this in mind when interviewing your doctor candidates. Most people will want a physician to be wagonmaster, but not all. I know several people who have nonphysicians as wagonmasters, though they almost always have physicians as "hired guns" on their team.

Some physicians are not yet comfortable with the idea of being on a patient's "healing team." Those who are open to this relationship realize the great advantages to both physician and patient. If the physician can accurately explain the benefits and risks of treatments, and the patient is actively involved in choosing one that fits best, it empowers the patient, more so than if the treatment is simply chosen by the physician. In this type of collaborative relationship, both the patient and the physician can choose whether or not they are comfortable with the treatment plan and choose whether or not to participate.

If a healing team makes sense to you but your physician won't hear of it, find one who will. If there aren't any such physicians where you live, consider moving, at least during your treatment phase. Of course, not everyone has this option, but you can always try to make up for deficiencies in your physician by utilizing other support systems. Going out of town for treatment can be expensive and can disrupt your support systems, so weigh the benefits and costs carefully. If you have a rare cancer, one that requires specialized treatments like marrow transplants, or one where there is considerable disagreement about treatment, it may be worth getting a major cancer center consultation to help guide your treatment choices.

Dealing with Uncertainty

One of the stresses that can confront you at this early stage is the uncertainty caused by conflicting opinions from experts. Variability in medical treatment is much more widespread than most people know. In his book, *Demanding Medical Excellence*, Michael Millenson examines how various problems are treated in the United States and finds remarkable differences, even in small geographic areas. One study asked primary care physicians in the Seattle area how they would diagnose and treat a simple urinary tract infection in a young woman—one of the simplest, most straightforward scenarios you can think of in medical practice. Remarkably, they got 137 different approaches from the 82 physicians interviewed. Clearly they got more than one response from some physicians, since there is more than one effective way to treat this simple condition.

While protocols in cancer medicine tend to be more standardized than in some other areas of medicine, there is still a good deal of disagreement and variability for treating many cancers. There are differences among geographic areas, between institutions, and even among oncologists in the same department in the same hospital. This reflects the fact that there is more than one way to treat cancer, and a certain amount of "art" as well as science is part of this process. Some of the art is fitting the treatment to the disease, but most of it is fitting the treatment to the person with the disease. That's why it's important to have a relationship with a cancer doctor in whom you feel confident.

When you find a doctor who treats you well, treat him or her well, too. David Spiegel of Stanford University, a psychiatrist who has done groundbreaking work in researching support for people with cancer, writes:

> We find that there are three keys to a good relationship with your physicians: communication, control, and caring. Be clear with your doctors about what you want from them. Participate in treatment decisions, and become informed about the choices you have. Find doctors who genuinely care about you as a person as well as treating your disease, and let them know how much you appreciate it.[2]

Balancing Activity with
Nurturance and Healing

Because there is often such a rush to gather information, get further medical testing, and get good opinions, the first weeks are often filled with activity, with no time to move into the emotional aspects of the experience. Anxiety levels can be so high during this period that you'll feel you cannot possibly rest until you know what's going to happen next. You may need to take medication to help you sleep and keep it together during the day, and that's fine. Do whatever helps you during this early period, including your healing imagery. Set aside some regular times during the day to use your relaxation and imagery abilities to help you stay in touch with yourself and your innate healing capabilities.

You may find it helpful to take a few days as a personal retreat after your diagnosis to come to terms with your initial reactions before you set out on the rest of the journey, or you may want to do this after gathering information about treatment options. While some cancers require taking action as soon as prudently possible, few demand true emergency action and it is often reasonable to take a few days to a few weeks if you need the time to sort things through and make your decisions.

The support of friends and family can be very important during this time. David Bresler, Ph.D., a psychologist and cofounder of the Academy for Guided Imagery makes this analogy about support: "Imagine that you are wandering alone in a strange part of town, it's dark and unfamiliar, and you see a pack of young men crossing the street toward you— are you nervous or scared? What if you had a friend with you—would you be a little less frightened? How about if you had six or ten friends with you? Would that make a difference?" Having people around who care for you, will fight for you, will research for you, and be there when you simply need to grieve or have company is a big help through this stage. The important thing is to know what is genuinely supportive for you and to be able to ask for the support you need—as well as for solitude when you need it.

Evaluating Support

When cancer strikes, any number of people may appear in your life whom you haven't seen in a while. Some will be helpful and supportive and some may turn out to be a drain on your energy and mood. Psychologist Jeanne Achterberg, one of the great mind-body researchers and authors, had a serious scare with cancer that went on for two years. At a conference sponsored by *Alternative Therapies* journal she talked about her experiences with support and described a welcome "support pie" of people in her life whom she found genuinely supportive—with sectors of intimate friends, loving supporters, trusted advisors, wise coaches, financial and logistical helpers, and just plain playmates. She also reported the challenges of dealing with a coterie of what she called "toxic support" characters—the "badgers," who urge you to "do something—anything or something specific, but do it right away!"; the "doom and gloomers," who already see you in the grave and can't help having long and sorrowful faces when they see you; the "projectors," who assume you are dealing with this the way they would—that their fears and beliefs are yours—and have no real interest in your feelings; the "users," who need you to take care of them and say something that will make them feel better; the misguided "New Agers," who ask, "What did you do so wrong as to give yourself cancer?"; and the "cancer fascists and fundamentalists," who think they know all the answers to having cancer—whether they come from medical, religious, holistic, or other perspectives.

It's important to decide for yourself how much time and energy you want to spend with various people during the different phases of your cancer treatment. You don't need to be rude to anyone, just take care of yourself. Leave an updated message on your answering machine, or ask one of your support people to field calls for you. I've had patients whose friends have set up websites to keep well-wishers current, without requiring the person fighting cancer to repeat the story whenever someone else is interested.

Support Groups

Support groups are often useful to people with cancer, and evidence shows they relieve stress and improve psychological functioning in many cancer patients.[3] At the same time, like everything else, support groups are not necessarily helpful for everyone all the time. Among the many types of support groups you have to find one that is genuinely supportive for you, at your stage, and with your concerns and beliefs. For some early diagnosed cancer patients, support groups can be scary, as you can find yourself with people going through different treatments and at various stages of illness, including some who may be very ill. You may also be somewhat more likely to find yourself with people who are not dealing well with their diagnosis. For this reason, many newly diagnosed patients stay away from support groups. The flip side, however, is that there are few better places to meet veterans of the war you are about to fight, and the right type of group can help you manage your stress and make better treatment decisions.

Some support groups are facilitated by a professional who helps keep people involved and helps the group address difficult issues with fairness and balance, and others are not. Some focus on information about specific types of cancer and are great sources of information about specific doctors and treatments—these can be particularly useful to you when you are first diagnosed. Others include stress and emotional management skills, like Dr. Fawzy's groups at UCLA, and many include self-hypnosis, relaxation, and guided imagery. All create a time and place to exchange information and express feelings among people sharing this challenge. Some groups, like those offered by the Center for Attitudinal Healing all over the world, focus on developing peace of mind, whatever happens.

The most effective support programs have a wide variety of groups to offer. One of the best I've ever seen is offered at the Ida and Joseph Friend Center in San Francisco, and directed by Keren Stronach, M.P.H. This center offers a tremendous variety of programs for patients at various stages; for different types of cancer; for family, parents, spouses, and children; and focusing on everything from healing to nutrition to finances. This variety makes a place for almost everyone, and Keren and her staff help people find a group that's good for them. If your community isn't lucky enough to have this kind of support yet, maybe starting one is a project for you when you get well.

Whatever is offered in your community, you may need to visit a few groups to see if they are for you. Ernest Rosenbaum is an oncologist who, with his wife, Isadora, a therapist, has been a leader in encouraging people with cancer to participate in their care. In their book *Coping with Cancer,* they give a simple guideline for evaluating support groups: "The best way to judge whether a support group is right for you is to attend a meeting. If you don't like it, don't go back."

Now let's move from outside resources to things you can do within yourself to reduce, relieve, or even transform the stress of having cancer.

Stress and Cancer

Stress is a term we apply to the response we have when we feel threatened, overloaded, or out of control. People newly diagnosed with cancer usually feel a good amount of all of these. We react to stress in different ways—some people feel it relatively directly and become more emotional, irritable, tearful, or anxious, while others react by increasing habits and behaviors that both signal stress and attempt to relieve it, such as overeating, or increasing alcohol, cigarette, or drug consumption. Still others develop physical symptoms—rapid heartbeat or skipped beats, shortness of breath, difficulty sleeping, loss of appetite, nausea, headaches, or neck and back pain.

Managing stress involves three major elements:

1. Changing the external situation
2. Changing the way you respond to the situation and/or
3. Changing the way you perceive or interpret the situation.

We've already talked about a few things you can do to begin to change the external situation: finding a good doctor and other helpers; reaching out for good, quality support, whether friends, family, professionals, or support groups; gathering information and making good treatment choices; and clarifying your goals and intentions. So now let's focus on some ways you can change the way you respond to the situation. Usually this involves both a shift in perspective and response, but let's focus on a simple shift in response first.

The stress response you may be feeling has certainly been triggered by an external event (your diagnosis), and your response is natural, but nonetheless you have an opportunity to alter your response internally and interrupt the stressful emotional and physiologic responses. This is where relaxation, meditation, self-hypnosis and guided imagery in their many forms come into play. Regular use of a relaxation technique like the one you learned in chapter 1 to create a healing place can help you in a number of ways.

The Benefits of Relaxation

I hope you have already experienced going to a place of peace and healing in your mind for relief and respite from the anxiety and difficult emotions you've been feeling. Regular and frequent visits to this place can be a tremendous aid in reducing the overall level of stress you feel. You will find that as you regularly relax, you will not only feel better while you do it but also reduce your overall level of arousal and stress and feel more in control.

The many benefits of relaxation have been known to many cultures for thousands of years, and have been rediscovered and validated by modern Western science. In 1972, Herbert Benson, M.D., and Richard

Wallace published a groundbreaking article in *Scientific American*, "The Physiology of Meditation."[4] Their research revealed that people trained in meditation demonstrated specific physiologic changes during and between meditations that were the opposite of what was seen in a stress response. During meditation the meditators had lower blood pressure, heart rate, breathing rate, and their cells used less oxygen than usual. They also cleared waste products out of their muscle tissues four to five times more effectively than they would even during sleep. Although the original research studied people trained in a specific form of meditation (Transcendental Meditation), later findings showed these effects to be produced by many forms of relaxation. Dr. Benson, now the long-time director of the Mind-Body Clinic at Harvard Medical School, came to call this the *relaxation response*. The guided imagery process you have already learned in Your Healing Place is a perfectly good way to induce this response.

The relaxation response is a specific physiologic state which is different than active waking or sleeping, and in that state it seems the body and mind are able to conserve energy and refresh and repair. If we look at the amount of time that so-called primitive cultures or primates like chimpanzees and gorillas seem to spend in just "hanging out," we can conclude that we are probably physiologically evolved to spend a fair amount of time in an awake but relaxed state. In busy modern lives our physiology rarely gets a chance to shift into this "refresh and repair" mode unless we specifically take time to make it happen.

Cultivating a regular practice of relaxation gives your body and mind a regular time to go into this rest, renewal, and repair state. In this state the body can use more of its energy for repair and healing.

Interrupting the stress response and inducing the relaxation response are major benefits of a regular relaxation practice, but there are others as well. First, you'll probably feel better while you are relaxing and in between, knowing that you can relax when you wish to. As you relax, you are likely to feel a bit more in control of yourself and better able to cope with the issues at hand.

In addition, relaxation teaches you to focus inside. And using guided imagery to relax not only makes this easier, it prepares you to use the imagery techniques you'll be exploring later.

The guided imagery processes you have already learned begin with relaxation and then move into imaging the healing responses within you, which usually results in you feeling more at ease. This probably derives from a combination of shifting your response as well as your perspective. Many people comment that after doing healing imagery they feel less like a helpless victim and more like a participant who has some potential in influencing outcome.

Evocative Imagery

I want to teach you another powerful imagery technique for shifting your response to your cancer diagnosis, a technique called Evocative Imagery.

In the beginning, you may be so devastated by the idea of having cancer that the consultations, opinions, and possibilities for treatment may leave you feeling weak, powerless, and scared. The idea of doing relaxation or healing imagery may seem remote at this time, since you may not feel particularly focused or powerful, or even able to conceptualize what healing would be like. You may need some emotional strengthening before you can begin to work with healing imagery of any kind. Evocative Imagery can be effective in helping you access your strength, your courage, and your determination. It can lift you out of a sense of helplessness and allow you to proceed in your best efforts to help yourself (or others.)

The Evocative Imagery technique for emotional shifting has been researched at Carnegie-Mellon University in Pittsburgh and was found to be extremely effective in helping people shift from one mood state to another. Learning that you can shift from helplessness to hopefulness at will is an empowering experience for anyone, especially if you are feeling overwhelmed by fear. The following story is a good example of how this technique can be used.

Emily, a nurse in her forties, had just been diagnosed with a recurrence of breast cancer when she came to see me. She could barely speak through her sobbing, but kept repeating, "I just don't know if I can do this again . . . I don't know if I can do it." She had been free of cancer for four years and had changed her life in many healthy ways after her initial diagnosis. She had improved her diet, clarified her personal goals, cleaned up some personal baggage through therapy, and since her treatment had been feeling better than she had in years. The recurrence was a shock and cruel blow, especially since she had "done all the right things" and had been feeling confident of her newfound good health.

Emily was willing to do imagery and I asked her what she felt she needed in order to be able to deal with the challenges that faced her. She quietly said, "I need strength . . . and courage . . . I don't know if I have the strength to go through this again."

I asked her to go back in her memory to a time when she did have the strength and courage she was missing now, and she chose to go back to a time twenty years earlier when her mother had been diagnosed with breast cancer. By asking her to imagine that she was there again, and to notice what she saw, heard, and felt, she was able to re-create the experience fairly vividly. As she described her mother sobbing and being terrified, as Emily had been at the start of the session, I asked her to pay attention to how she felt. She said that she was calm, clear, and encouraging to her mother. She felt scared and sad, but also felt a sense of strength and confidence that they'd be able to take whatever steps they needed to take to deal with this. I invited Emily to notice where she felt these qualities of strength and confidence, of calmness and clarity, and over a few minutes, to imagine that she could feel them very strongly in her body, and she did. She was able to experience these qualities in herself and when she opened her eyes, much calmer and more composed, she said, "You know, I do have the strength I need, I just couldn't get to it."

This is often the case when you have cancer. With so much fear and stress you lose access to these strengths at a time when you need them most. Evocative imagery allows you to reconnect with your own resources and begin to use them effectively. Emily still had a recurrence of cancer to deal with. She still had to evaluate different treatment options, make difficult decisions, and go through some potentially unpleasant treatments. She still had to deal with uncertainty about her prognosis and a host of other challenges that cancer can bring, but now there was a difference. She was back in touch with her strength, her courage, and her clarity. And when she lost touch with these qualities, which she periodically did over the next few months, she had a way to get back in touch with them. She found evocative imagery to be a useful tool to help her reconnect with her strength and she practiced it frequently, especially over the first few weeks after her diagnosis of recurrence. When I saw her a few weeks later, she remarked, "You know, this type of imagery is kind of like emotional bodybuilding, isn't it? The more I do it the stronger I feel, and the easier it is to do."

The comparison is a good one, since imagery and its effects generally get better and more effective with repetition. It's a mental process that has physical effects. As with most skills, the results you get will improve with practice.

YOUR EXPERIENCE WITH EVOCATIVE IMAGERY

Before moving into your inner world, take a few moments to think about a particular quality that you'd like to feel more of right now. It might be strength or courage, like Emily, or it might be calmness, patience, confidence, peacefulness, or any other quality you'd like to feel. This is a process you can use over and over so don't worry about the first quality you choose—you won't wear your imagination out no matter how much you use it. In fact, you'll strengthen it, as well as the qualities you evoke as you repeat the process.

Sometimes the way you want to feel involves more than one quality. It's fine to have two or maybe three qualities to focus on in any one session, but more than that tends to dilute the effectiveness of the process.

You can probably think of having more courage, clarity, and strength and use that trio of qualities as your focus, but you may not have as much success trying to feel calm, courageous, confident, patient, humorous, philosophical, and ferocious at the same time.

To prepare to explore with evocative imagery, write about the following in your Healing Journal:

How are you feeling right now?

What quality or qualities would you like to feel more of in yourself?

Recall and describe a time you felt these qualities in yourself.

If you haven't had that experience, describe a time you observed these qualities in someone else.

What do you imagine it would be like to experience these qualities more powerfully in yourself?

How would you think? feel? act?

How would it help you to express more of these qualities right now?

When you are finished writing, get comfortable and take about twenty to thirty undisturbed minutes to explore the following evocative imagery process. We'll begin once again with breathing, relaxation, and going to your place of healing.

Evocative Imagery

Take a comfortable position and let yourself begin to relax in your own way . . . let your breathing get a little deeper and fuller . . . but still comfortable . . . with every breath in, notice that you bring in fresh air, fresh oxygen, fresh energy that fuels your body . . . and with every breath out, imagine that you can release a bit of tension . . . a bit of discomfort . . . a bit of worry . . . and let that deeper breathing and the thoughts you have of fresh energy in and tension and worry out be an invitation to your body and mind to begin to relax . . . to begin to shift gears . . . and let it be an easy and natural movement . . . without having to force anything . . . without having to make anything happen right now . . . just letting it happen . . . just breathing and relaxing . . . breathing and energizing. . . .

Come back to taking a few deeper breaths whenever you feel like relaxing even more deeply . . . but for now, let your breathing take its own natural rate and its own natural rhythm . . . and simply let the gentle movement of your body as it breathes allow you to relax naturally and comfortably . . . almost without having to try. . . .

And noticing how your right foot feels right now . . . and how your left foot feels . . . and noticing that just before you probably weren't aware of your feet at all . . . but now that you turn your attention to them, you can notice them and how they feel . . . and notice the intelligence that is there in your feet . . . and notice what happens when you silently invite your feet to relax . . . and become soft and at ease . . . and in the same way noticing the intelligence in your legs and releasing your legs . . . and letting the intelligence in your legs respond in their own way . . . and noticing any release and relaxation that happens . . . without having to make any effort at all . . . just softening and releasing . . . and letting it be a comfortable and very pleasant experience. . . .

And you can relax even more deeply and comfortably if you want to . . . by continuing to notice the intelligence in different parts of your body and inviting them to soften and relax . . . and noticing how they relax . . . and you are in control of your relaxation and only relax as deeply as is comfortable for you . . . and if you ever need to return your awareness to the outer world you can do that by opening your eyes and looking around and coming fully alert . . . and if you need to respond to anything there you can do that . . . and knowing that you can do this if you need to . . . you can relax again and return your attention to the inner world of your imagination. . . .

Inviting the intelligence of your low back, pelvis, and hips to release and relax . . . and your abdomen and midsection . . . and your chest and rib cage . . . without effort or struggle . . . just letting go but staying aware as you do. . . .

Inviting the intelligence in your back and spine to soften and release . . . in your low back . . . mid-back . . . between and across your shoulder blades . . . and across your neck and shoulders . . . the intelligence in your arms . . . and elbows . . . and forearms . . . through your wrists and hands . . . and the palms of the hands . . . the fingers . . . and thumbs. . . .

Noticing the intelligence in your face and jaws and inviting them to relax . . . to become soft and at ease . . . and your scalp and forehead . . . and your eyes . . . even your tongue can be at ease. . . .

And as you relax, let your attention shift from your usual outer world to what we can call your inner world . . . the world inside that only you can see, hear, smell, and feel . . . the world where your memories, your dreams, your feelings, your plans all reside . . . a world that you can learn to connect with . . . that can help you in many ways on your journey. . . .

And imagine that you find inside a very special place . . . a very beautiful place where you feel comfortable and relaxed, yet very aware . . . this may be a place that you have actually visited at some time in your life . . . in the outer world or even in this inner world . . . or it may be a place that you've seen somewhere . . . or it may be a brand-new place that you haven't visited before . . . and none of that matters as long as it is a very beautiful place, a place that invites you and feels good to be in . . . a place that feels safe and healing for you. . . .

And let yourself take some time to explore this place . . . and notice what you imagine seeing there . . . all the things you see . . . and how you see them . . . don't worry at all about how you imagine this place as long as it is beautiful to you and feels safe and healing . . . and notice if there are any sounds you imagine hearing . . . or if it is simply very quiet in your healing place . . . notice if there is a fragrance or aroma that you imagine there or a special quality of the air . . . there may or may not be, and it's perfectly all right however you imagine this place of healing . . . it may change over time as you explore it, or it may stay the same . . . it doesn't matter at this point . . . just let yourself explore a little more. . . .

Can you tell what time of day it is? . . . or what time of year it is? . . . and what the temperature is like? . . . how you are dressed? . . . take some time to find a place where you feel safe and let yourself get comfortable there . . . and just notice how it feels to imagine yourself there . . . and if your mind wanders from time to time, just take another deep breath or two and gently return your attention to this beautiful and healing place . . . just for now . . . without feeling the need to go anywhere else right now . . . or do anything else . . . just for now. . . .

And now think about the quality or qualities that you'd like to feel more of in yourself . . . silently name them or say them aloud if you wish . . . and let your mind take you to a time when you felt these qualities in yourself . . . and imagine that you are there once again . . . and notice where you are . . . and notice what you are doing . . . and who you are with, if anyone. . . .

Take some time and notice the details . . . notice what you see as you look around . . . and notice what you hear . . . let yourself be there now in your own way . . . and notice if there are any smells or aromas . . . and how it feels to be there. . . .

And if there was never a time when you felt these qualities in yourself, imagine what it would feel like if you did feel them . . . now . . . you might imagine someone else you have noticed these qualities in . . . someone you know or a historical figure . . . and then imagine that those qualities are in you now. . . .

Pay special attention to the feelings of the qualities you came to experience again . . . notice how it feels to have them within you . . . and notice where you feel them most strongly in your body . . . gently scan with your attention through your body and notice if these feelings seem to center anywhere . . . if they are stronger in one area than another . . . in your face or head? . . . in your chest? . . . your abdomen? . . . pelvis? . . . arms? . . . legs? . . . anywhere else? . . .

And as you imagine yourself there again, feeling the qualities you desire to cultivate again . . . notice how your body posture is as you feel those qualities within you . . . and notice how your face feels as you allow the feelings of those qualities to be there . . . how do you imagine your voice is as you talk with the awareness of these qualities in you? . . . and how do you move? . . .

If you are comfortable with it, imagine that you can allow the sense of these qualities to grow a bit in you . . . to gently grow a bit stronger and expand . . . stay relaxed and comfortable and imagine that the feelings begin to grow so that they fill your whole body . . . as if every cell of your body were touched by the feelings that go with these qualities . . . let the feelings develop, like a photograph develops. . . .

Imagine that the feelings radiate out from wherever they are centered . . . radiating out in all directions, like the light from the sun . . . filling your body with this quality or qualities . . . imagining that you feel the quality all the way down your legs to the bottoms of your feet . . . and all the way down your arms to the palms of your hands and tips of your fingers and thumbs . . . and filling your face . . . and touching the very deepest core of your being . . . and all your organs . . . and bones . . . and muscles . . . and all the other tissues and cells in your body that are healthy . . . and filling each of them with this quality . . . and just be with that for a little while . . . soaking up those qualities like a sponge . . . and becoming saturated with them . . . naming them again, silently or out loud. . . .

Then, if you like, imagine that you have a knob or control as you do on a radio or television, and you can turn up the strength of the qualities just as you'd turn up the volume on a radio, and imagine turning up the volume so that the feelings of the qualities overflow your body for a foot in every direction . . . and see how that feels. . . .

And if you like you can turn it up even stronger . . . so you fill the space around you for several feet in every direction . . . and fill the room around you with the feeling of those qualities . . . and the town you are in . . . and the whole world if you like . . . just imagine turning it up as far as you like . . . and don't turn it up any more if you feel at all uncomfortable at any point . . . and you can turn it back down to where it feels comfortable to you at any time . . . bigger isn't necessarily better . . . just adjust the feeling to whatever is most pleasant to you right now . . . it's like listening to a radio when you are the only one in the room . . . whatever is most comfortable to you right now is exactly right . . . adjust the strength of the feeling to be most comfortable . . . and enjoy that for a few minutes more . . . and feel free at any time to adjust it either way. . . .

And you can let those feelings stay with you as long as you like and even bring them back with you when you decide to return your attention to the outer world. . . .

And taking all the time you need. . . .

And when you are ready to return your attention to the outer world, silently express any appreciation you might have for finding a special healing place within you . . . and for being able to use your imagination in this way . . . and for being able to connect with your own inner strengths and helpful qualities . . . and when you are ready, notice the qualities within you, and as you allow all the images to fade . . . you can bring this feeling back with you if you like . . . and you can always connect with it and strengthen it by recalling it in this way . . . and gently bring your attention back to the room around you and the current time and place . . . and bring back with you anything that seems important or interesting to bring back, including any feelings of comfort, relaxation, or healing . . . and when you are all the way back, gently stretch and open your eyes. . . .

And take a few minutes to write or draw about your experience.

Debriefing Your Experience

After you've written or drawn what you want to remember, ask yourself these questions and write some more in response.

What qualities did you want to experience?

What memory took you back to them?

What did you notice as you imagined yourself experiencing that time again?

How was it for you to feel these qualities within yourself?

How do you feel after this process?

Do you feel any different than before?

What did you learn from this experience?

What level of intensity was most comfortable for you to experience?

How do you think you will use this process in the future?

What other thoughts or questions do you have about this experience?

Shifting Your Perspective

The third major movement for reducing stress is considering whether your perspective and interpretation of the events that are causing you stress is the truest, or only true, interpretation of the facts.

Perspectives form the truth for us in many situations—the five blind men examining the elephant are the classic model for this. One says, "It is as big around as a barrel" as he hugs the elephant's leg, while another, holding the tail, exclaims, "No, no, it is a like a broom." The one holding the trunk describes it as a large hose, the one examining the tusk says it's a long tree branch, and the one holding the elephant's ear says it's like a big palm leaf. To the extent they don't know they are not grasping the whole elephant, they can get entrenched in their positions. They could all learn more about the elephant and get a more comprehensive view by sharing their perspectives, or even better, trading positions.

Perspective is important in dealing with cancer. It can determine how you will respond to your options, treatments, setbacks, and victories. So let's look at some common perspectives on cancer and some alternatives.

TOXIC PERSPECTIVES ON CANCER

Ideas about cancer and its treatment can be potent inhibitors or potentiators of treatments and of healing. The best example of this is probably the effect that expectations can play in both increasing and decreasing adverse reactions to chemotherapy. Studies have shown that a third of nausea and vomiting in response to chemotherapy is anticipatory—people get sick just thinking about their treatment. This is an effect of imagination and expectation, and may perhaps be called "unguided imagery," or "misguided imagery." Although chemotherapy is strong medicine, and can have adverse effects, negative expectations set up people for an even worse time than they need to have. Developing fear and dislike about the treatment amplifies negative reactions and often results in not being able to tolerate or complete a full dose of treatment. When you don't complete your treatment, it doesn't work as well as it might, so this is more than a simple inconvenience—it can make the difference in whether or not your treatment is effective. Perspectives and expectations have real effects that can augment or weaken treatments and treatment responses.

An idea that I believe is most daunting in the medical approach to cancer is the concept that the tumor has all the power. Oncologists will often say that the determining factor in outcome from cancer is the cell type and stage of tumor. We type the tumor cells by identifying what kind of cells they are (breast, lung, colon, etc.) and assign a stage to the illness by determining whether it has spread from its original location. Typing and staging is an important process that allows us to be more precise when using the powerful modalities we bring to cancer treatment. It also allows us to better differentiate when certain treatments are likely to be useful and when that is less likely.

However, correlating outcomes with tumor type and stage alone ignores the potential healing influence the person with cancer can have, an element in outcome that has unfortunately been relatively ignored in cancer research. As far as I know, there is no current way to quantify healing potential, and perhaps that's one reason it's been overlooked. Scientists are fond of things that can be measured and quantified, and tend to ignore the many other things that don't conveniently yield to these processes. It's not that healing potential cannot be quantified, just that it's more difficult than researching simple interventions like medicines.

The fact that people have variable responses to cancer treatments at all stages of treatment is well documented, and while the majority of patients with a certain type of tumor at a certain stage may have a certain response, a substantial minority will always have either a worse or better outcome than the average. This alone tells us that factors other than the tumor determine what happens to an individual, and it is rationale enough for seeing what you can do to improve your prognosis.

The interaction between the agents of disease and the resistance or vulnerability of the "host" (that is, you) has been recognized for ages in medicine but tends somehow to get lost in the way we commonly think about, talk about, and even treat people with illnesses. Here's a common example: in cold and flu season someone with a bad cold sneezes repeatedly in a crowded elevator containing ten people. About four of those people will soon come down with a cold. If the virus that is associated with the cold is especially powerful, maybe five or six of them will get sick. If the virus *causes* the cold, why doesn't everyone get sick? The obvious answer is that some people are more vulnerable to the virus. Their resistance or immunity is decreased for whatever reason—sleep deprivation, excessive stress, too much alcohol, other illness, or poor nutrition being common factors. At the same time, those who didn't get sick had enough resistance or immunity to fend off the virus without it being able to invade.

Given the above scenario, why do we say "viruses cause colds and flu"? Clearly they are involved, but they are only one factor. A virus by itself is not sufficient material out of which to make a human cold— you also need fertile ground in which the virus can grow—so it's the combination of the disease factor and host resistance that determines what happens. It's reasonable to assume that a similar process, perhaps involving different mechanisms, is at work in how people fend off cancer. We may not know the exact factors, but it certainly bears looking at the most reasonable ones (sleep, nutrition, mood, stress, mind) while the search goes on. So that's what we're focusing on here—the mental/emotional/spiritual aspect of *resistance*, the "ain't necessarily so" aspect of your response to cancer and its treatment.

There are many well-documented cases of people who have

unexpectedly survived Stage 4 cancers, and of people who have unexpectedly succumbed to what are generally treatable cancers, in spite of getting good medical treatment. What accounts for this variability? We don't know yet. Perhaps as pathologists type tumors more accurately we will find variations that help us get better with treatment, but I suspect there will always be variability in patient response. The difference in response is either in the patient or in one other possibility—it's in the "mystery." The mystery is what you might call God, destiny, fate, karma, or life, but whatever you call it, it is all those things that happen in life that do not seem to be under our control, whether good or bad, desirable or undesirable.

If it's in the mystery, what can you do? You can pray to it, petition it with rituals, images, thoughts, desires, wishes, and intentions. Who hasn't found that at least sometimes it seems to respond favorably to our prayers? And who hasn't found that sometimes it doesn't? I once asked a priest friend why God didn't answer all prayers. He laughed and said, "God does respond to every prayer, but not always in the way you desire."

We all deal with the mystery in our own way. Our attempts to use our minds to influence it through imagery is akin to a type of prayer. The main difference is to whom you are addressing your messages—are you communicating with an external diety or your internal healing mechanisms? In either case, the process is similar. We ask for help, for guidance, for strength, and for healing from whatever we think has the power to deliver these things. Whether the help that comes originates outside or within ourselves is a matter of personal belief, philosophy, and experience. I personally prefer to issue the call for assistance to all the powers that be and be glad of any responses—whether they seem to be from the inside or outside.

So while your cancer specialists work to help you eliminate your tumor, keep working within yourself to better understand and stimulate the healing responses that you—or whatever you call the mystery—can bring to the effort.

PERSPECTIVES ON IMAGERY

So far you've had a chance to explore three imagery processes that can help you shift your response and perspective in varying degrees. Let me now share a fourth process that is powerful for reducing fear, gaining strength, and navigating your way through your journey with cancer. It involves inviting an image that can represent the immense healing intelligence within you and finding out how you can support each other. We can call this figure an Inner Healer, a figure that is wise, caring, and powerfully healing. The Inner Healer is a variation on a technique we usually refer to as the Inner Advisor process. The difference is that we ask that the Inner Healer has great knowledge and ability in healing.

It's not really far-fetched to imagine you have such intelligence within you. Just being alive means you have inherited the healing wisdom that life has accumulated over several billion years. Think about it. How did you get here in the first place? Whether you think of it as nature, life, God, genes, or DNA, something inside you is intelligent enough to take one single cell and grow it into you, from whatever you've been eating or drinking all your life, whether it's asparagus and goat cheese or Gatorade and Tostitos. This is not mysticism, it's embryology.

Whatever it is that grants us life began by taking a single microscopic cell in your mother's uterus, one that had joined with a single microscopic cell from your father, and made it divide in two. Both those cells are identical, as far as any scientist can tell—they have the same structure, components, ingredients, genes, and so on. Then they divide and there are four identical cells. Then eight at the next division, then sixteen, and so on. All these cells are still identical as far as we can tell.

By the time you got to where you were a still microscopic ball of cells, all identical, a line of cells on one side of the ball started to become different (the process is technically called differentiation) and a darker streak formed that we call the neural streak. This line of cells will multiply and expand and eventually form your skin, brain, spinal cord, and all your nerves. Soon afterward, the ball folds in on itself and ends up being a ball with a tube running through its center.

The cells that line this tube grow and differentiate according to genetic and chemical signals to become your digestive tract, your heart and blood vessels, your lungs, liver, spleen, kidneys, and other organs. The cells between the outer and inner layer become your muscles and connective tissues (tendons and ligaments) and your bones. All these things develop in a highly coordinated series of movements, so that as an embryo you go through various stages where you look like a tadpole, a fish, a chicken, a pig, a monkey, and finally emerge looking generally like Winston Churchill. Then, of course, you keep growing and learning, changing dramatically though your infancy, childhood, adolescence, and adulthood. Nobody understands how this happens, but it happens reliably and repetitively, so that over 95 percent of all births are of normal children.[5]

During your life I am sure you have fallen ill, or injured yourself in some way. The great majority of the time you probably healed and recovered from whatever illness or injury you suffered. If you've had a serious illness or injury before, you may not have ended up exactly the way you were before, but you can bet that your body, and the life that flows through it, did everything possible to mend the broken bones, heal the wounds, eradicate the infections, or eliminate the poisons. Without belaboring this point, it's obvious that without powerful systems of healing and repair, none of us would have lived long enough to be able to get cancer in the first place.

But wait, you say—in spite of these healing abilities something has now gone wrong in you. Somehow your defenses are down, or your life's ability to organize your body and keep it differentiated has failed—otherwise you wouldn't be faced with cancer. That's precisely why we want to focus on not only destroying cancer cells but on nourishing and strengthening the internal communication systems that allow the body to maintain itself in good health.

The Inner Healer process is a variation of a method that has been used for ages in many different approaches to healing. So-called primitive and shamanic cultures would journey into the spirit world looking for a powerful animal ally to help fight the demons or spirits that were believed to be involved with causing the disease. In traditional Tibetan medicine, prayers would be offered to a specific manifestation of divinity called the Medicine Buddha. Patients would be encouraged to center themselves, invite this powerful deity into their awareness, and ask it for help with their healing.

In every culture, people pray when they are ill—in thousands of different ways, with different words and different rituals, to different perceptions of God. The one difference between prayer and guided imagery has to do with whom you think you are addressing when you are using your mind in this way. Someone praying is appealing to a higher power, a god, or gods and goddesses, a spirit of some kind that is perceived and thought of as being external and separate to the person. With guided imagery, we use imagery, the coding language of the mind, to influence physiology, to stimulate healing, to create relaxation, and to connect with our own wisdom and strengths. I don't think that these processes are mutually exclusive; use them as you feel most comfortable and confident. You can use imagery as an element of prayer or as a method of self-healing, or both. I don't see why we can't simply appeal to the powers that be, whether they are internal or external, and thank them when we notice them working on our behalf.

In the imagery process that follows, you will be invited to relax, go to your special place of healing, and imagine you are there with a figure that is both wise and kind, but also powerful and ferociously protective of you, your Inner Healer. Imagine that your Inner Healer knows a great deal about you and about healing, a figure that can help guide, protect, and help you heal. You may have both an Inner Advisor and Inner Healer; in fact, you may have an army of healers and advisors by the time you've worked with this process for a while. You can call on your unconscious mind for whatever information or help you need—pay attention to how it responds and you will frequently be pleasantly surprised.

For the purposes of helping to reduce or resolve stress, an Inner Advisor may help by comforting you or by showing you a different viewpoint on issues that are problematic for you, while an Inner Healer image may be more directly involved in stimulating physical healing. Don't get caught up in semantic differences. I recommend exploring with the script and letting the figure come as it will, exploring with it to find out how it can be most helpful to you.

Some people think the idea of an Inner Healer or Advisor is kind of odd, but it really isn't. Think about how you make important decisions in your life. When you have a really important decision and it's hard to make rationally, what is it that you ultimately listen to? Most people say they have a "gut feeling" or that their intuition tells them. What tells you when you're on the right track or not? How reliable has that voice been throughout your life? Most people tell me that when they listen to this particular voice (though they usually don't really hear a voice) it almost always works out for the better for them, and when they ignore it they often pay for it. That's another way to identify and think about your inner guiding figures. They are not exactly a conscience and certainly not a critic—they are friendly guides that help you when you're in need and don't know what to do.

Preparing for Your Meeting with an Inner Healer

In this imagery process, you'll relax, go to your special place of healing, and then invite an Inner Healer or Inner Advisor to meet you in that inner place. Your Inner Healer or Advisor is friendly, wise, powerful, protective, and knows a lot about healing. You may imagine this figure in any way—it may come to mind as a person, animal, spirit, religious figure, plant, cartoon, movie character, or any other form. It might come as you have pre-imagined it, or it might surprise you. As with all these imagery processes, let yourself explore for a while to see why any particular image came to mind. As long as the figure you imagine is friendly and caring, see what it has to offer you.

Although it's important to be receptive when using this imagery technique, you do not have to agree in advance to act on anything you learn. It's best to take some time to consider whatever you learn, analyze it, and then make decisions about what to act on, just as you would after consulting with any other advisor or consultant.

As you immerse yourself in your inner world, you may find different perspectives about situations that are stressful to you. Your Inner Advisor or Healer can give you input from their perspectives, but you'll always bring back what you've discovered and consider it in the "clear light of day" before making any decisions that might affect you or others you love or care for. Treat the experience like any consultation you might seek, as a trusted source of caring and wisdom, and consider carefully what comes back to you.

Now take some time to clarify what you want to focus on when you meet your Inner Healer or Advisor, and what question you most want to ask. Write in your Healing Journal before you journey to meet your Inner Healer. Answering the following questions will be useful:

Have you ever had an experience with an Inner Advisor or Inner Healer, where something inside you guided and helped you resolve a difficult or stressful situation, whether you imagined a figure or not?

If not, what do you imagine a wise guide would have told you at that time?

What guides you in a pinch? When you've had difficulty making an important decision, what is it that ultimately you listen to?

What do you imagine your guide would look like if it took a form you could imagine conversing with?

What would you like to ask your Inner Advisor or Inner Healer when you meet with it?

Sometimes your questions will change as you get more deeply relaxed, and that's fine. Moreover, this can be just the beginning of what often turns out to be a long-lasting relationship, so you don't need to cover everything the first time you meet. Meet with your Inner Healer the same way you'd meet with anyone you thought could be helpful to you.

Meeting with Your Inner Healer

Take a comfortable position and let yourself begin to relax in your own way . . . let your breathing get a little deeper and fuller . . . but still comfortable . . . with every breath in, notice that you bring in fresh air, fresh oxygen, fresh energy that fuels your body . . . and with every breath out, imagine that you can release a bit of tension . . . a bit of discomfort . . . a bit of worry . . . and let that deeper breathing and the thoughts you have of fresh energy in and tension and worry out be an invitation to your body and mind to begin to relax . . . to begin to shift gears . . . and let it be an easy and natural movement . . . without having to force anything . . . without having to make anything happen right now . . . just letting it happen . . . just breathing and relaxing . . . breathing and energizing. . . .

Come back to taking a few deeper breaths whenever you feel like relaxing even more deeply . . . but for now, let your breathing take its own natural rate and its own natural rhythm . . . and simply let the gentle movement of your body as it breathes allow you to relax naturally and comfortably . . . almost without having to try. . . .

And noticing how your right foot feels right now . . . and how your left foot feels . . . and noticing that just before you probably weren't aware of your feet at all . . . but now that you turn your attention to them, you can notice them and how they feel . . . and notice the intelligence that is there in your feet . . . and notice what happens when you silently invite your feet to relax . . . and become soft and at ease . . . and in the same way noticing the intelligence in your legs and releasing your legs . . . and letting the intelligence in your legs respond in their own way . . . and noticing any release and relaxation that happens . . . without having to make any effort at all . . . just softening and releasing . . . and letting it be a comfortable and very pleasant experience. . . .

And you can relax even more deeply and comfortably if you want to . . . by continuing to notice the intelligence in different parts of your body and inviting them to soften and relax . . . and noticing how they relax . . . and you are in control of your relaxation and only relax as deeply as is comfortable for you . . . and if you ever need to return your awareness to the outer world you can do that by opening your eyes and looking around and coming fully alert . . . and if you need to respond to anything there you can do that . . . and knowing that you can do this if you need to . . . you can relax again and return your attention to the inner world of your imagination. . . .

Inviting the intelligence of your low back, pelvis, and hips to release and relax . . . and your abdomen and midsection . . . and your chest and rib cage . . . without effort or struggle . . . just letting go but staying aware as you do. . . .

Inviting the intelligence in your back and spine to soften and release . . . in your low back . . . mid-back . . . between and across your shoulder blades . . . and across your neck and shoulders . . . the intelligence in your arms . . . and elbows . . . and forearms . . . through your wrists and hands . . . and the palms of the hands . . . the fingers . . . and thumbs. . . .

Noticing the intelligence in your face and jaws and inviting them to relax . . . to become soft and at ease . . . and your scalp and forehead . . . and your eyes . . . even your tongue can be at ease. . . .

And as you relax, let your attention shift from your usual outer world to what we can call your inner world . . . the world inside that only you can see, hear, smell, and feel . . . the world where your memories, your dreams, your feelings, your plans all reside . . . a world that you can learn to connect with . . . that can help you in many ways on your journey. . . .

And imagine that you find inside a very special place . . . a very beautiful place where you feel comfortable and relaxed, yet very aware . . . this may be a place that you have actually visited at some time in your life . . . in the outer world or even in this inner world . . . or it may be a place that you've seen somewhere . . . or it may be a brand-new place that you haven't visited before . . . and none of that matters as long as it is a very beautiful place, a place that invites you and feels good to be in . . . a place that feels safe and healing for you. . . .

And let yourself take some time to explore this place . . . and notice what you imagine seeing there . . . all the things you see . . . and how you see them . . . don't worry at all about how you imagine this place as long as it is beautiful to you and feels safe and healing . . . and notice if there are any sounds you imagine hearing . . . or if it is simply very quiet in your healing place . . . notice if there is a fragrance or aroma that you imagine there or a special quality of the air . . . there may or may not be, and it's perfectly all right however you imagine this place of healing . . . it may change over time as you explore it, or it may stay the same . . . it doesn't matter at this point . . . just let yourself explore a little more. . . .

Can you tell what time of day it is? . . . or what time of year it is? . . . and what the temperature is like? . . . how you are dressed? . . . take some time to find a place where you feel safe

and let yourself get comfortable there . . . and just notice how it feels to imagine yourself there . . . and if your mind wanders from time to time, just take another deep breath or two and gently return your attention to this beautiful and healing place . . . just for now . . . without feeling the need to go anywhere else right now . . . or do anything else . . . just for now. . . .

And allow yourself to become aware of anything here that feels healing to you . . . it may be the beauty . . . it may be the sense of peacefulness . . . it may be the temperature, or the fragrance, or a combination of all the qualities that are here . . . perhaps you have a sense of what's sacred to you and what supports you in your life . . . it doesn't matter what you find healing here . . . or whether you can even identify it specifically . . . but let yourself experience whatever healing is there for you . . . and simply relax there . . . and know that while you relax, your body's natural healing systems can operate at their highest efficiency . . . without distraction . . . and without needing to be told what to do. . . .

(Pause for 10 seconds)

And when you're ready, invite an image to appear of a figure that is wise, caring, and knows a great deal about healing . . . allow the image to form more clearly . . . and accept the image that comes into your mind . . . it may be a figure new to you, or a familiar figure, and either is fine . . . as long as the figure is friendly and helpful . . . it may come in just about any form . . . as a person you've known or someone new . . . another sort of living creature . . . a religious figure, even a cartoon character . . . it may come as a presence or a light . . . simply allow it to be what it is for now and take a few moments to carefully observe the image. . . .

It's important to notice whether you feel comfortable in the presence of this figure . . . and notice whether the image seems kind, and caring . . . notice whether you can feel its caring for you . . . and notice, too, if it seems wise . . . and notice any healing qualities it has . . . take some time to really check it out. . . .

If you don't feel a sense of caring and safety with this image, then send the figure away and imagine instead that you are there with an image that is friendly, helpful, and healing . . . an image you do feel comfortable with . . . and that feels like an Inner Healer. . . .

Imagine now that your Inner Healer is willing to help with the issue you have come to discuss . . . take some time to notice how this image appears, and notice the qualities that it has . . . imagine that you can communicate with this figure and ask its name . . . imagine that it can respond to you in the way you can understand. . . .

Your Inner Healer may speak directly to you, or communicate with you in some other way that you can understand . . . be open to what you receive as you begin to communicate with your Inner Healer now, and be sure to thank it for coming . . . and when you're ready, let it know about the situation you have come to get help with. . . .

Let your Inner Healer know what you'd like help with and allow it to respond to you . . . allow yourself to be receptive to what it has to communicate. . . .

Your Inner Healer may offer you guidance or information, or it may show you something about healing . . . or it may do something with you that feels healing . . . just notice how it responds. . . .

Pay careful attention to any guidance or healing that comes . . . and be receptive to any healing rituals or actions it offers you . . . give this some time . . . if you haven't already, ask it if there's anything specific it would advise you to do to ease your journey through cancer and to help you heal . . . and pay careful attention to its responses. . . .

You can continue to communicate with this figure at any time by simply returning to your safe inner place and inviting your Inner Healer to come into your awareness, so you can discuss the issues and questions you have or ask help with your healing . . . paying careful attention to how it responds and what it has to share with you. . . .

When you bring any advice back to your outer life, please consider it again carefully and make whatever decisions are right for you . . . you can decide whether or not to act on any of this advice, or to come back and continue the creative conversation with your Inner Healer, until you find solutions that work well for you . . . and if it has done something that feels healing within you, bringing that memory and feeling back with you as well. . . .

And when it seems right to you, thank your Inner Healer for coming to be with you today . . . and take a few moments to review what has happened in this experience . . . notice especially anything you want to make sure to bring back with you when you return your attention to the outer world . . . whether it's an action you want to take or a feeling you have within you. . . .

(Pause for 15 seconds)

What did you receive from your Inner Healer today? What did you learn or observe about healing? Is there anything you've learned that you want to make sure to bring back with you when you return to your outer world?. . .

When you are ready, take your leave from your Inner Healer . . . in whatever way seems appropriate to you . . . remembering that you can come back to this inner place anytime you want to rest, to relax, to focus on healing, or to ask for help from your Inner Healer. . . .

(Pause for 30 seconds)

And when you are ready, allow all the images to fade and go back within . . . knowing that healing continues to happen within you at all times . . . and gently bring your attention back to the room around you and the current time and place . . . and bring back with you anything that seems important or interesting to bring back, including any feelings of comfort, relaxation, or healing . . . and when you are all the way back, gently stretch and open your eyes. . . .

And take a few minutes to write or draw about your experience and what you've learned.

Debriefing Your Experience

Once you've written and drawn what you want to remember about this experience, consider the following questions as you expand on your understanding of this process:

Draw your Inner Healer and whatever seemed significant about this experience.

What was your Inner Healer like?

How did it appear to you, and what qualities did it have?

What did you ask, and how did it respond?

How did it feel to be with this figure?

What guidance did it give you?

Did it do anything to you or with you?

How did that feel?

What did you learn in this session?

Is there anything you'd like to ask for or do with your Inner Healer the next time you meet?

How do you imagine you could use this connection to help you achieve your healing goals?

Reviewing the Options for Reducing Stress

You've now been exposed to four processes that can help you reduce fear and stress, marshal your mental strengths, and boost your healing responses. Which seem most useful to you now? Use whichever process is most helpful as frequently as you need to in order to stay in touch with yourself and your strengths. Some people are most comfortable with a special healing place, while others feel best imagining a ferocious cancer elimination process going on inside. Some find great comfort and courage from their Inner Healers, while others don't relate to that. Trust yourself and your intuition. Go easy on yourself and use what works for now—different approaches work better for different people, and also at different times, so don't struggle with any of them—use what helps the most in any given situation.

Again, make at least one, preferably two or three times a day to put other things aside and practice your ability to relax, go inside, and work with some form of healing imagery. The more you do it, the more benefits you will receive.

Summary

- Stress and emotional turmoil are the biggest causes of distress in the early weeks of a cancer diagnosis, so learning to manage these well is especially helpful.
- External support from a good doctor, family, friends, and support groups is helpful if well selected. Evaluate what the best support is for you.
- Stress management has three components: changing the situation; changing your response to the situation; and changing your perspective on the situation. The Evocative Imagery and Meeting with Your Inner Healer scripts in this chapter can help you with all three components.

4

❖

Why Is Imagery Important?

Do you remember your dreams or gain direction from them? Do you know how to daydream? Can you get lost in a good book or in a movie? Do you cry during movies or commercials? Have you ever seen shapes in clouds? Have you ever prayed? Have you ever had an imaginary companion or a guardian angel? Have you had experience with hypnosis, self-hypnosis, meditation, relaxation techniques, biofeedback, or shamanic journeying? Are you interested in any of these practices?

If you answered yes to any of these questions you are a good candidate for using guided imagery to help you through your experience with cancer.

The first question most people have about guided imagery and cancer is: "Can I cure my cancer through it?" To put this into perspective, here are some similar questions: "Will tennis lessons guarantee me the club championship?" "Will an M.B.A. guarantee me a successful business experience?" "If I marry the high school football hero will I live happily ever after?"

Just as the answers to these questions depend on many factors, whether you recover from cancer also depends on many factors, some known and many unknown. Known factors include the type of tumor you have, its stage, its aggressiveness, its location, the effectiveness of treatments for it, your general health status, your selection of treatments, your willingness and ability to follow through with treatments, where you are treated, and by whom you are treated. Yet even all of these factors can't predict except in statistical terms how likely recovery is for you. Many people who were not supposed to survive cancer have beaten the odds, with virtually every type and every stage.

The purpose of using your mind well is to increase the likelihood that you will have the outcome you desire. In addition, imagery can be helpful to you in many ways, whether it cures your cancer or not. Here's a partial list of reasons to learn to use imagery, even if you completely disregard its potential for curing cancer:

+ Imagery is comforting and tremendously stress relieving.
+ Imagery stimulates your immune system.
+ Imagery is enjoyable.
+ Imagery is better than worrying.
+ Imagery can show you things about yourself and life that are good to know.
+ Imagery can relieve pain.
+ Imagery can prevent or reduce nausea from chemotherapy drugs.
+ Imagery can prevent complications and pain after surgery.
+ Imagery can reduce distress during radiation therapy.
+ Imagery can expand your awareness of your body, feelings, mind, and spirit.
+ Imagery can help you resolve or come to terms with inner conflicts.
+ Imagery can help you access your strength and courage.
+ Imagery can connect you to your creativity and problem-solving abilities.
+ Imagery can enhance your intuitive abilities and help you with decision making.

+ Imagery can help you clarify and refine your communications with others.
+ Imagery can help you connect with your own spirituality.
+ Imagery can help you find peace of mind.

In addition, there is reason to believe that through all of the above, and through other mechanisms we don't yet know about, imagery may well help you overcome your illness and return to good health.

What Is Imagery?

Imagery is a natural way that humans store and process information. It's an efficient way to store memories and work with future possibilities. Like all higher brain functions, imagination is a mystery, but it's not mystical. It's simply a way of thinking that uses sensory information for processing. Imagery consists of thoughts that can be seen, heard, smelled, tasted, or sensed in some way in your mind.

We have images of people we know and people we've never met, events we've experienced and events we'd like to experience, places we've been and places we have read about, seen on television, or perhaps just dreamed up. Memories, dreams, fantasies, plans, illusions, and lies all involve imagery. Art, whether visual, musical, or conceptual, all involves imagery: it is the language of poetry, painting, music, myth, and drama.

Since imagery is a way of thinking, there are countless ways to use it to fight or cope with cancer. You can use imagery to relax, to escape stress, to relieve pain, to stimulate blood flow, immunity, and other healing mechanisms of the body, to generate creativity, to help make decisions, to resolve inner conflicts, and to process and manage emotions.

The challenge is learning how to use your imagination skillfully, rather than just using it to worry yourself silly.

The first skill most people learn with imagery is using it to relax, and if you've done any of the imagery scripts in the previous chapters you've already learned to do that. Regular interruption of chronic stress with relaxation "mini-vacations" or visits to your place of healing can sustain your energy, positive mood, and abilities to cope with the challenges your illness and its treatment may bring.

Beyond relaxation, imagery can be used to stimulate your immune system and alter blood flow to areas of the body, two major mechanisms of healing. You began to imagine this in Your Healing Place imagery and you'll learn to do more with healing imagery in chapter 5.

Imagery can stimulate your creativity and help you find solutions to difficult problems. An imaginary conversation with a wise and helpful guide (an Inner Advisor or Inner Healer) will often provide creative and useful solutions to difficult problems, and if problems are not soluble, they provide internal support.

If you explored the technique of "Evocative Imagery" in chapter 3 you learned that imagery can be used to cultivate qualities you'd like to have more of, such as courage, patience, tolerance, humor, concentration, self-confidence, or others that can support you through your cancer treatment. Whether for relaxation, problem solving, healing, or self-development, learning to use your imagination skillfully can be one of the best investments you'll ever make with your time.

Imagery is a natural way that we think, but few of us have ever had any real education in learning how to use it for healing. Before I get too technical, you might want to make sure you've explored some imagery. If you haven't yet experimented with any of the scripts in the previous chapters, I recommend that you do the first process, "Your Healing Place," on page 20 and see what a simple imagery technique can do for you. Then come back here if you'd like to read more about imagery.

◈

Imagery can be thought of as one of the brain's two major coding languages. The one we are most familiar with is called the *sequential* information processing system, which uses words and numbers. Words and numbers let us think about things in the abstract, but don't have direct sensory equivalents. Like the number 4. You can imagine four apples or four horsemen and you can imagine the number 4 itself as you see it on a blackboard or printed page, but you can't imagine the quantity "four" itself, because it is an abstract concept. The same with "insurance" or "health" or "love." Words and numbers allow us to name and quantify things, however, so they are useful in logical thought.

Imagery, however, is the language—or coding system—utilized by a *simultaneous* information processing mode of thinking, which tends to perceive how things are related as part of a larger whole. It lets us look at the tapestry into which the details of a situation are woven. It can help us grasp the bigger picture. The relationships represented by imagery, like the relationships in a tapestry or painting, may not be logical, but they are still meaningful and make their own kind of emotional sense. Imagery is closely tied to our emotions, and emotions can directly and indirectly help or hinder us in our efforts to heal.

Emotions are important in mind-body healing, not only because they motivate us to action, but because they also produce physiologic changes in the body by varying patterns of muscle tension, blood flow, respiration, metabolism, and biochemistry. Modern research in psychoneuroimmunology (PNI) points to the emotions as key modulators of chemicals secreted by the brain, gut, and immune systems. In addition to being a rapid route to insight, understanding, and motivation, imagery can have direct physiologic consequences and effects. In the absence of competing sensory cues, the body tends to respond to imagery as it would to a genuine external experience.

Imagery has been shown in numerous research studies to affect almost all major physiologic control systems of the body, including breathing, heart rate, blood pressure, metabolic rates, digestive functions, sexual function, and perhaps most important, immune system response.

A review of articles investigating whether imagery could affect immune response revealed that the vast majority of twenty-two such studies showed significant positive results.[1] They demonstrated that people doing imagery aimed at stimulating the immune response against cancer or chronic viral illnesses increased not only the numbers of circulating killer cells (the immune cells specifically charged with eliminating cancer cells) but increased their aggressiveness when encountering an abnormal cell or virus. The immune system responds to chemical signals generated by the brain, the gut, and other immune cells. These chemicals (interferons, interleukins, and others) can heighten or reduce the activity level and aggressiveness of the immune defender cells, can increase or decrease the production of new immune cells, and can help direct the cells to areas where they are most needed. Since the brain is a major source of these chemical signals, why not use it to turn your immune system on to high alert and high level activity against cancer?

The level to which immune responsiveness is increased with imagery is significant. I would say that if there were a drug that did the same thing, especially if it had the complete lack of side effects that imagery has, nearly every cancer patient in America would be on it, or the doctor would risk a malpractice suit. A great deal of research is taking place in institutions around the world on the uses of interferons and interleukins for stimulating the immune system. The trouble is, when they are injected at very high levels, as they usually are for medical purposes, they are difficult for the patients to tolerate—they can cause intense flu-like symptoms, debilitating fatigue, and serious depression. Conversely, when the system is stimulated by imagery, there are no adverse side effects. Any side effects actually tend to be positive—a greater sense of calmness, empowerment, and feelings of wholeness.

Because of the three-way relation that imagery has to thoughts, emotions, and physiology, we might well consider imagery to be the Rosetta stone of mind-body interactions.

A Brief History of Imagery in Healing

Imagery can be considered the oldest and most ubiquitous form of medicine, since it is involved in all healing rituals and interactions. From the first time a human (or even a prehuman primate) cried out for help for an ailing companion, and perhaps prayed for their health, imagery was used in healing. Healing traditions in nearly all premodern cultures were always done in the context of prayer and ritual, which are, at least at one level, forms of imagery. Even today, while religious rituals are rarely part of modern medicine, both the patient and the doctor have expectations, hopes, and fears, and thus the imagination plays its role, however unconsciously, in every healing transaction.

The traditional rituals of various cultures all have a certain level of efficacy or they wouldn't persist, and though we may attribute these therapeutic benefits to "placebo effects," they are *real and measurable* effects with important implications for our understanding of the healing process.[2] While I do not think that all the benefits of imagery are caused by the placebo effect, I do think that the benefits' mechanisms are probably intimately interrelated, and so the term placebo merits some attention.

Placebo effect is widely misunderstood in medicine. It is often interpreted to mean "nothing happened" or that the patient "simply thought they were better," but placebo effects are real and measurable effects on healing, whether from physical or mental illness or symptoms. The placebo effect accounts for more than half of the response of all major pain relievers, including morphine and other narcotics.[3] In fact, when strong placebo responders (meaning people who get good pain relief from sham injections) are then injected with drugs that block the effects of opiates, they lose their placebo response to pain.

That indicates that when they believed they were getting a medication for pain relief, their own brain secreted opiatelike substances (endorphins) to relieve the pain.

The point here is that placebo is a real effect. The case could well be made that we change its name to the "mind-body healing effect." If we can be "tricked" into healing by being given sham treatments, why then shouldn't we be able to turn on that response within ourselves? I believe we can, and imagery seems to be an important code language for doing just that. The human brain is the world's greatest pharmacy. It makes chemicals that relieve pain, stimulate immunity, relieve nausea, and control most of the trillions of functions going on in our bodies all the time. UCLA pain expert David Bresler, Ph.D., says that imagery is the key to this pharmacy, and that's one reason we'll spend so much time learning to use it. But first let's return to the history of imagery in healing to put this all in context.

Shamanic healers in many ancient cultures enter a trance state during which they claim to journey to the spirit realm to have direct discourse with the spirits or gods that affect health or illness. In shamanic cultures, the spirit world is considered to be a real world, more real than the world we live in, which is considered a dream world.[4] The spirits are considered to be autonomous, external, and separate from us. We do many of the same things the shamans do in guided imagery, but we usually consider the images to be aspects of our own inner self. In truth, we really don't know what's within us and what's outside us in these realms, but as doctors and patients, this isn't really important. Our concern is whether these approaches are helpful in healing. My years of experience with this in practice have made me quite certain that they are.

Some Native American medicine men painstakingly create detailed and ornate sand pictures by slowly placing individual colored grains of sand to create an image that depicts how the illness came about and how it can be healed. In the paintings you can see the patient, the medicine man, and the spirits believed to be involved. The patient, often after fasting and praying for some time, watches this hypnotic process of sand painting unfold and is often profoundly affected by it. There may be more to it, but this is at the very least a potent form of guided imagery.

In India, the ancient Hindu sages believed that images were one of the ways that the gods sent messages to people, and they developed a wide range of specific imagery techniques as an integral part of yogic practice.[5]

Mind-body healing practices such as chi gung and its derivatives have been an integral part of traditional Chinese medicine for thousands of years.[6] Tibetan culture has perhaps developed imagery as a healing art more profoundly than any other. Focused concentration on specific colors, sounds, deities, and images is prescribed for specific conditions and is felt to have great healing power. Receptive meditations are also used, such as appealing to a deity called the Medicine Buddha for guidance.[7] This may well reflect a healing archetype also revealed in the Aesclapian ritual of dream incubation or in your imagery dialogue with a caring wisdom figure like your Inner Advisor or Inner Healer.

Healing rituals, whether considered to be prayer or guided imagery, continued to be an essential part of medicine and healing during the birth of Western culture. Esoteric teachings of Judaism encouraged the practice of *kavanah*, a state of peaceful concentrated awareness, and utilized this state to focus on images within the cabalistic model of healing.[8]

In ancient Greece, the dominant healing model at the time of Hippocrates considered the imagination to be a vital organ. In their model, the senses took in reality, subtracted its matter, and took the remainder into the psyche (soul) where it formed images. Some of these images stimulated emotional reactions which, in turn, moved the four humors, which were thought to mediate balance and health in the body. If you substitute the term peptide molecules for humors, this model is quite current in light of what we know from psychoneuroimmunology research.[9]

Galen, the Roman physician who was the dominant influence on Western medicine for a thousand years, considered the imagination to be a critical element in both creating and healing illness, as did Paracelsus, a fifteenth-century physician best known as the father of chemical medicine. Paracelsus, one of the most celebrated and innovative physicians of his day, went so far as to say that "the spirit is the master, the imagination the tool, and the body the plastic material."[10]

Medicine was dominated by and limited by religious restrictions in the West until the French philosopher René Descartes declared the body to be machinelike and independent of the mind and spirit.[11] This alleged separation, though inaccurate, freed physicians and scientific thinkers to explore the body as part of the natural world and paved the way for tremendous advances in our scientific understanding of physiology and pathology. In the enthusiasm for the physical discoveries that followed this release, the power of the mind received little attention until it dramatically resurfaced in the person of Anton Mesmer.

Mesmer was an Austrian stage performer who literally entranced Parisian and European culture with his dramatic healing rituals. Dressed in flowing purple robes, Mesmer would pass his hands around an ailing person's body, affecting its "animal magnetism" until the subject would faint or fall into a trance state. Numerous healings, often of hysterical ailments (but sometimes of well-documented physical conditions) led to great notoriety and fame. Mesmer's cures were investigated by the prestigious French Academy of Sciences, which insightfully declared the beneficial effects to be real but attributed their source to be the "influence of the inspired imagination."[12]

James Esdaille, a British surgeon practicing in India, performed major operations utilizing Mesmer's techniques as the sole anesthetic. Another contemporary surgeon, James Braid, coined the term hypnosis to describe a relaxed state in which people seemed to be hypersuggestible and reported it to be remarkably effective in relieving pain and healing difficult illnesses. At about the same time, Jean Charcot, a French neurologist and teacher of Freud, utilized this approach as a treatment for conversion symptoms including blindness and paralysis.

This "psychological cure" became the basis for Freud's fascination with the unconscious mind and led to the development of his psychological theories and practices.[13]

Carl Jung, the eminent Swiss psychiatrist, believed that imagery was as close to the unconscious as one could get, or that it may even *be* the unconscious mind directly revealing itself. Jung employed a method he called active imagination as a means of gaining insight into his client's unconscious process. He would invite his patients to relax and focus their attention on their symptoms, and describe the images that came to mind. He reported that "at first, the client tends to watch the images with some fascination, as if at the theater, but sooner or later it dawns on them that they are being addressed by something intelligent."[14] This idea, that your imagery is produced by an inner intelligence, is the basis for our later explorations of imagery dialogue techniques, where you can imagine conversing or communicating with various images, be they of your body, your illness, your immune system, or your inner wisdom and learn things of value in your healing journey.

Roberto Assagioli, an Italian psychiatrist and contemporary of Freud and Jung's, developed a spiritual psychology called psychosynthesis in response to what he felt was the unbalanced approach of psychoanalysis. Assagioli, like Jung, believed that the unconscious not only held repressed drives and unacceptable urges (as Freud postulated), but that it was also the source of creativity, altruism, empathy, inspiration, and many other higher human attributes. He utilized and taught guided imagery as an effective path to awareness.[15]

In America, at the turn of the twentieth century, leading psychologists such as William James made extensive use of imagery, but as psychology attempted to become a science, a laboratory-based behavioral model became dominant and images or any other "unmeasurable" mental contents were considered unfit for academic investigation for over fifty years. In 1964 a landmark paper by R. R. Holt, "Imagery: The Return of the Ostracized," was published in the *American Psychologist*, signaling a resurgence of interest in this area.[16] Leading psychologists such as Jerome Singer, Arnold Lazarus, Akhter Ahsen, and Joseph

Shorr began once again to develop, research, and write about imagery applications in psychology and mind-body medicine. Anees Sheikh, professor of psychology at Marquette University, greatly helped to stimulate professional interest in imagery through his leadership as editor of the *Journal of Mental Imagery* and organizer of a number of seminal national and international conferences.

Imagery again came to light in medicine in the late 1960s with the startling reports by radiation oncologist O. Carl Simonton and his then wife, psychologist Stephanie Simonton, of unexpected longevity in cancer patients following the use of imagery and visualization to stimulate immune response. The Simontons taught their patients simple relaxation and imagery techniques they learned from Silva Mind Control, a commercial course utilizing mental imagery for enhancing performance, relaxation, memory, and healing.

Although the Simontons' work stirred a great controversy in medicine, little clinical research was done in this area until the late 1980s. The development of psychoneuroimmunology as a field of study finally encouraged researchers to cross disciplinary boundaries to study the effects of the mind on physiology and healing. Although this research is just beginning, many studies have already validated the Simontons' early hypothesis that people can stimulate their immune response through imagery. As reviewed earlier, several studies indicate that psychosocial and mental interventions extend the lives of cancer patients. Psychologists Jeanne Achterberg and Frank Lawlis, working with the Simontons, helped to formulate some of the earliest research in this area, developing the Image CA, a rating scale of imagery drawings by cancer patients. They found that certain aspects of the imagery work may predict clinical outcome, and developed similar scales and imagery interventions in the areas of chronic pain, diabetes, and spinal injuries as well.

A seminal influence for me was osteopathic physician/author Irving Oyle. A masterful physician, Oyle explored the profusion of new approaches to healing that blossomed in the early 1970s with a clinician's eye for effectiveness. Oyle derived the technique of dialoguing with an imaginary figure of wisdom and compassion (Inner Healer or

Advisor) from his readings of Jung and his personal experiences with Silva Mind Control.

My longtime colleague and partner, David Bresler, Ph.D., innovated the multidisciplinary holistic approach to pain at UCLA in the early 1970s and, inspired by Oyle, Simonton, and others, began to research and develop imagery applications in medicine and psychology. In response to mounting requests, he and I developed formal clinical training programs for health professionals in 1983. With ongoing feedback from thousands of postgraduate students, we tested, expanded, redefined, and codified the methods we had learned from our studies of Jungian psychology, psychosynthesis, Gestalt therapy, Ericksonian hypnotherapy, object relations theory, humanistic psychology, and communications systems theory. Over time, this experience gave birth to Interactive Guided Imagery^sm, an extremely powerful yet remarkably safe therapeutic approach for mobilizing the untapped healing resources of the mind.

In 1989, we founded the Academy for Guided Imagery to provide in-depth training to practicing health care professionals, to raise public and professional awareness about the potential benefits of imagery, and to support research, the dissemination of information, and professional communication in the field. We recruited an interdisciplinary faculty, set standards for certification, obtained professional accreditation, and created the 150-hour professional certification curriculum that the Academy offers today.

How Imagery Relates to Hypnosis, Meditation, and Other Mind-Body Approaches

Since imagery is a natural language of the unconscious—a coding language intimately related to our feelings, experiences, memories, and visions—it is involved in nearly all mind-body approaches to wellness and healing. Other prominent modalities in mind-body medicine include relaxation techniques, meditation, hypnosis, biofeedback, and body-mind approaches such as yoga, tai chi, and chi gung. When you closely examine what actually happens in each of these practices, you find it almost always has to do with imagery—either focusing on it or letting it go.

Relaxation techniques are the most widely used, easily learned, and generally useful mind-body techniques available because stress is often a significant factor in illness and health-related issues. Stress can be considered part of almost any illness, in that it can cause the illness, amplify the distress involved, or can itself be caused by the illness. Reducing stress allows one to feel better, regain some sense of control, and concentrate the body's energy on healing. As discussed in chapter 3, stress is largely a problem of imagination, and the easiest and most effective overall technique I have found for relaxation is the one that I hope you have already done—going to a peaceful, safe place inside and taking a 5- to 20-minute daydream vacation.

No matter which relaxation method you use, it will involve two things—a way to distract your focus from worrisome thoughts (products of your imagination) and a new focus on thoughts that are neutral or actively calming and relaxing.

There are many forms of meditation, but they almost always involve concentrating your attention on either a neutral or meaningful focus—a word, image, external object, your breath, or whatever is occurring at the time. Meditation tends to create a physiologically relaxed state and helps develop peace of mind. Some forms of meditation are connected to particular religious belief systems, but many others are not and are perfectly compatible with any belief system. Part of why meditation is so useful is that it teaches people to focus their attention on something other than their habitual worries. In essence, it is a way to begin freeing your mind from its attachment, fascination, and perhaps even addiction to fearful and worrisome thoughts. It is also a way to free yourself from a runaway imagination, a first step toward learning to use your imagination skillfully.

Biofeedback uses sophisticated, sensitive physiologic monitors to amplify the reactions your body is having in response to your thoughts.

By being able to see, hear, or otherwise experience changes the body makes in response to thoughts, it is often possible to gain control over physical functions normally out of conscious control. Biofeedback is a convincing experience for most people who explore it, as it is quite enlightening to see how quickly and sensitively the body responds to thoughts. Biofeedback has particularly exciting applications for victims of stroke and head injury, for problems of incontinence, and for alcoholism and other addictions. When we get to the point where we can measure immune responsiveness quickly and noninvasively, we may even be able to develop biofeedback techniques for stimulating immunity. Nearly all the mental processes that biofeedback therapists teach their patients are imagery related, and the biofeedback shows you exactly how your body responds to these thoughts, at levels that are at first difficult to feel. If you have any doubt that your mind affects your body, I'd strongly encourage you to seek out a qualified biofeedback therapist and have at least one session so you can see for yourself.

People who work with guided imagery often have beginning concerns or questions about its relation to hypnosis, a much misunderstood phenomenon. Guided imagery and hypnosis are different, although there is much overlap between the two. Hypnosis refers to a state of relative relaxation in which your attention is highly focused. Hypnotic states happen naturally, like when you are watching movies or television or when you are thoroughly absorbed in doing something like driving long distances (highway hypnosis).

The tendency to go into a hypnotic state varies between individuals, although most people are capable of focusing in this way. Many people think of hypnosis as a mystical interaction where the hypnotist "takes over" people's minds and can make them do things they wouldn't normally do. This impression derives largely from stage and television hypnosis acts, which are often truly amazing and appear to produce just these results. Stage hypnotists use a variety of techniques to be successful, such as selecting audience members who are ready to do whatever they're asked. This is often accomplished by performers watching the audience for those who are laughing at their jokes, nodding their heads, or even leaning toward them when they move or gesture. These are people with high hypnotizability who are favorably disposed toward the hypnotist. Once such people are called onstage, the pressure to comply with suggestions mounts and is amplified by the disorientation and anxiety most inexperienced people feel onstage. All this results in them being highly likely to do what the hypnotist asks, after whatever ritual they are told will put them into a "trance."

The truth is, they are already in a trance state and unconsciously responding to the stage hypnotists' suggestions before they are selected. This is all very entertaining, but therapeutic uses of hypnosis are quite different. Many professionals who use hypnosis teach their patients to create a self-hypnotic state that they can use for their own benefit. This state of highly focused, concentrated attention often occurs spontaneously when you focus on your breathing, relaxation suggestions, and images that come to mind. Technically, hypnosis is the state of awareness you have when you are relaxed and focused. Emmett Miller, a prominent psychiatrist who has been a pioneer in using therapeutic hypnosis for healing, has appropriately called hypnosis a state of "selective attention."

When you are learning to relax and focus on your imagery, you will be in what can be called a self-hypnotic state, although you could also call it a state of relaxed, concentrated attention. With guided imagery you will learn to put yourself into and bring yourself out of this state of relaxed, concentrated attention at will, and use it to help yourself. It's a state you naturally go into when you get lost in a good book, a movie flies by, or you drive for a while and wonder how you got where you ended up. It's not dangerous and nobody else will control your mind. In fact, learning to use this state of relaxed, focused concentration along with your imagery puts you even *more* in control of your mind than you were before.

With the guided imagery skills I'll teach you, the imagery content and suggestions for solutions to your challenges come from within you. The relaxed focused state makes it easier for you to be able to pay attention to your imagery, which is subtler than the many stimuli and demands presented by the outer world.

Interactive Guided Imagery[sm] (IGI) is a specific way of using imagery that has been developed by the Academy for Guided Imagery. The academy teaches health professionals to work with this process and creates self-help programs and materials for the public. IGI is particularly effective in helping you develop insight into your potential roles in your own recovery and in helping you to use your inner resources most effectively. In this form of imagery, you are led to explore and work with personal imagery about your illness and healing, clarify any issues that may be involved, and learn to use the mind to support your healing. The methods you'll learn here that involve imagery dialogue are based on IGI principles in that there will be opportunities to become aware of and interact with your own images. I believe that these are ultimately the most powerful images to work with because they are obviously the most personal, they come from your own inner database of experiences and memories, and thus are most relevant and meaningful to you in your healing journey.

You already used IGI principles when you were invited in chapter 1 to go to a place of healing inside and when you took the opportunity to imagine your own Inner Healer. While I invited you to relax and create a mental space for this, the images of your healing place and the healing you imagine are uniquely yours, and because they are uniquely yours, I believe they are likely to be more powerful than images that someone else suggests or gives you.

For many people, a place of healing is outdoors in nature, but for others it's in a church, in a childhood home, or in an imaginary temple of healing. For most people, the healing place is calm and peaceful yet powerful, though I have patients who imagine their healing place as a place of great power and energy, fueled by thunder and lightning and wind that they soak up and use for eradicating cancer. With most people, the imagery of healing includes fighting, destroying, and eliminating cancer cells, but for others it involves imagining that the cells are returning to their previously healthy state. I encourage you to explore for a while to find imagery that feels right and powerful for you.

You may come across ideas, images, or pictures that appeal to you and that you include in your own imagery, and that's just fine. Just as you learn more and more about anything that interests you, or is important to you, the same will happen with your use of imagery. You may notice that your imagery for healing changes or evolves on its own over time, even without interjecting new material on a conscious level. It will become even more powerful and refined as you work with it.

In the next chapter we'll look in more detail at creating healing imagery that's personal, powerful, and meaningful for you.

Summary

- Imagery is a natural way our brains store and process information.
- Imagery involves sensory-based thinking.
- Imagery can show us the "big picture" perspective and has powerful emotional and physiologic effects.
- Imagery is one of the oldest forms of healing and has been used in almost every era and tradition of medicine in history.
- Imagery is involved in nearly all forms of mind-body healing, including meditation, biofeedback, and hypnosis.

5

Stimulating Healing

The spirit is the master,
imagination the tool, and
the body the plastic material.
—Paracelsus

When you decide to focus on recovery and begin to construct positive healing visualizations and imagery scenarios, it is a way of committing to a direction and intention. Focus on your target as you would aim for any bull's-eye. You are much more likely to hit it than if you aren't aiming at it—or don't even know it's there!

Your body is a complex organization consisting of trillions of cells. Any organization that we know of, be it a business, a nonprofit, a team, a club, or even a family, operates more smoothly and easily if it has a vision to guide it. If an organization has a vision of what it wants to be or what it wants to do, and if that vision is effectively communicated throughout the organization, it greatly increases the likelihood that the organization will accomplish what it wants to accomplish. If there is no clear vision, the organization will be much more vulnerable to outside influences and the winds of change. That's one way to look at healing imagery—it gives all of you—body, mind, and spirit—a vision to follow.

Some years ago I was on a search committee to find a new head for the school my daughters attended. We asked the various candidates what they saw as the prime job of the head of the school. There were several interesting answers, but the winning candidate simply said this: "The job of the head is to repeatedly articulate the vision." Of course, a head has many other duties, mobilizing support and resources, resolving conflicts and disputes, hiring and firing, managing resources, etc., but always in the light of the vision. It's the vision, articulated and communicated, that organizes the decisions and movement of the organization.

Our bodies' cells, digesting, metabolizing, carrying out their specialized functions, are working together in an intricately coordinated way. We take this organization for granted until we learn that something is not working right, or something threatens our abilities, our freedoms, and even our existence. Then the treatments that we bring to bear have as their aim the return to a balanced, healthy, self-repairing and regulating community. While most of this is built into us, and beyond our ability or need to control, it can be influenced by what we think, feel, and how we act. Your head can repeatedly "articulate the vision," in this case the vision of healing, and in doing so increases the likelihood that the organization will follow suit.

You already started creating images of healing in chapter 1. Since then, you've probably gotten more input and understanding about your illness, its treatment options, your healing capabilities, and what other healing approaches can contribute. I hope you have also experimented with some of the other imagery techniques offered, and that your imagery of how healing happens has already changed and developed. In this chapter we'll concentrate on updating, refining, and amplifying the effects of such images, a process that may continue throughout your healing journey.

First, let's examine more closely the common questions that people have about this process, and then you'll have a chance to once again go to your place of healing and work with your current images of healing.

In thirty years of teaching imagery to tens of thousands of people, these are the questions I have heard most frequently about healing imagery for cancer:

+ What are the best images for healing?
+ If I can help myself with imagery, does that mean I've somehow caused my cancer?
+ How can I make my imagery more powerful?
+ How can I make my imagery more tangible?
+ What if I have trouble imagining healing at all?
+ How can I imagine healing when my tests show the cancer is still there?
+ What aspects of physical healing can imagery potentially influence?

Once we look at the issues these questions raise, I'll invite you to explore an extended guided imagery process that you can continually use to refine and update your healing imagery practice.

What are the best images for healing?

I feel strongly that your own unique imagery is the most powerful since it arises from your own internal understanding of the process. Since healing is an unconscious process, an image that springs from your unconscious mind is likely to be more "custom fit" and effective than an image that someone else prescribes. Imagery, after all, is the natural language of the unconscious, and healing is an unconscious process. By inviting an image of healing and allowing yourself to explore what comes, you invite the unconscious to inform your healing. This is my opinion, however one that hasn't yet been proven or even studied.

It's important to work with your imagery of healing to make it as congruent as possible with how you experience yourself in this journey. At the same time, you'll want to periodically explore your view of yourself, your healing abilities, and your treatments, if they are going to stay powerful and current.

A man in a prostate cancer support group once approached me and said, "You know, I have trouble imaging an aggressive immune system response to my cancer because it doesn't seem that that is what really controls this cancer. There is no evidence that poor T-cell responses make any difference in prostate cancer." I said I thought he was probably right, but that the body has other ways of protecting itself against cancer growth that we don't yet understand and others that we haven't even yet identified. I recommended that he let his imagery represent his body's "cancer defense systems," which made sense to him and allowed him to imagine his body containing and eliminating cancer in new ways.

Clearly, the body has mechanisms for identifying and destroying cancer cells, but when we look at patients who are immune-suppressed, like transplant patients and HIV patients, they don't generally develop most cancers more than the average population. They can and do develop certain blood cancers (lymphomas) but not solid tumors like lung, breast, prostate, or colon. So there are other factors involved in eradicating cancer cells or preventing cancer growth and we don't know what they all are or how they work. That's why I think you should let your imagery represent the body's ability to eliminate cancer, however you imagine it and leave the details up to the unconscious healing abilities you have. We don't yet understand all the ways a body protects itself from or heals from cancer.

IMAGE AS GUI

I sometimes think of images being what the computer people refer to as GUIs—graphical user interfaces. The picture or graphic you see on your computer screen is a symbol for a process that can happen, not the process itself. The little garbage can icon that I throw files into to dispose of them isn't really a garbage can, but it tells me how to throw away files without having to understand complex computer programming language. It makes it simple: I drag a file to the garbage can and the computer "knows" what I want it to do and it does it. That's how I think of healing imagery—the image conveys your desire and intention to the unconscious, which is the part of you that knows how to carry out your directions. The actual healing is far beyond our current understanding, and yet we all heal all the time throughout our lives.

To find what's right for you, try out different forms of imagery and see what feels most right and powerful. I provide you with a number of different approaches in the imagery scripts, and you can see what resonates most strongly.

If I can help myself with imagery, does that mean I've somehow caused my cancer?

Of course not. Just because you may be able to help yourself with your mind doesn't mean that you gave yourself this disease. Just because a batter gets a home run doesn't mean he made himself strike out three times before that. If you donated some money to charity, that doesn't mean you made other people poor beforehand. If you find a cure for cancer, it doesn't mean that you caused it in the first place, with your mind or anything else.

Nevertheless, it's very common that people with cancer feel guilty or ashamed for having this disease, and blame themselves for the trouble, expense, and grief they feel they are causing their family and friends. This shame and guilt is something that not many people talk about, except in support groups, with therapists, or perhaps close friends or spiritual advisors.

People with cancer (this is also true for people with other chronic illnesses such as arthritis, multiple sclerosis, chronic pain, etc.) often feel "different" than others, even alien. Cancer carries with it some of the feelings and associations that leprosy once did: it can feel unclean and threatening, and some people even have fears that it can be contagious. While you may feel modern and above such things, your primitive feeling responses, in search of reasons, may welcome the idea that you did something wrong to bring this about. Many people fear loss of control more than any other single threat—and finding a reason for the cancer, even if the reason is a seemingly terrible one, like feeling that you caused it or that God is punishing you, at least takes it out of the realm of the unknown.

Psychologically, cancer may even serve to balance your internal books about guilt and blame. In a strange way, it can be a relief to be found guilty, convicted, and sentenced. Thus guilt, blame, and shame find a psychological niche in cancer and its treatment. But it's just as important to know there are other ways to feel more in control and have more say in what happens to you. There are other ways to accept responsibility for mistakes you've made, or even venal sins you may have committed, and ways to seek genuine forgiveness and penance for such things.

One way to get a perspective on guilt and blame is to turn the whole mind-body cancer issue on its head. Could you give yourself cancer if you wanted to? Certainly lifestyle habits and choices can move you into groups much more likely to have cancer, but even assiduous and persistent involvement in these pursuits wouldn't guarantee that you'd develop cancer. You could smoke cigarettes, drink to excess, never eat fruits or vegetables, and nurse grudges for years without being guaranteed of developing cancer. You'd have better odds, of course, but no guarantee. So don't waste your energy blaming yourself for having cancer—use your energy instead to focus on what you can do to help yourself heal.

The question still before you is: What will you do now? Where will you go and what will happen if it's up to you? And what are you willing to invest, personally, in terms of time and energy, attention and intention, in order to get to where you say you want to go?

Guilt, blame, and shame are common in all of us. Nobody avoids mistakes in this life. Nobody fails to hurt others, even, or maybe especially, those who are closest to us. It's the nature of the game—but what do we do with those hurts and those regrets? Do we use them to make us better people, or to keep us feeling unworthy of anything but punishment? If so, this can be a significant deterrence to wholehearted healing. What can you do about it? Coming to terms with and reducing the emotional energy stuck in guilt, blame, and shame, can release energy to be channeled into healing.

James Pennebaker is a psychologist who was consulting in the Texas prison system when he noticed an interesting phenomenon. Observing many polygraph (lie detector) tests, he noticed that suspects frequently broke down and confessed to their crimes after a period of lying and trying to cover them up. He also noticed that after they confessed, even to horrible crimes, knowing that they would then face certain punishment, the polygraph machine showed that physiologically they relaxed. Once the jig was up they were able to let down.

Of course, the power of getting something off your chest, and the relief that often comes when you've told someone else something that is weighing on you, is well known to psychologists, priests, and friends alike. Pennebaker decided to see if he could separate the effect of confession from other aspects of therapy and counseling. He took two matched groups of college students and invited the experimental group to sit down and write about the worst things that had ever happened to them or that they had ever done in their lives. The instructions were to keep writing, without editing or censoring, about these events, people, feelings, and whatever else they thought about for twenty minutes. They repeated this exercise four days in a row. The control group also wrote for twenty minutes but on topics not involving feelings or personal material.

Pennebaker found that the students who had written about their difficult experiences and their feelings had half the visits to the Student Health Service as the control group. They also felt better about themselves psychologically. Pennebaker has done similar studies, published in the *Journal of the American Medical Association*, that have shown beneficial results lasting over six months in measurements of health in people with rheumatoid arthritis and asthma.[1] Writing about experiences and feelings had widespread beneficial effects on physiology, both mentally and physically.

Even if you don't feel guilty or to blame for your illness, you may want to spend some time with Pennebaker's exercise. Take twenty minutes to write about the worst things that have happened to you or that you have ever done and all the feelings and thoughts that come to mind about these events and how they affected you. This includes your cancer diagnosis. Don't edit and don't censor—you don't need to share these notes with anyone unless you choose to. Pennebaker noticed that for the first two days some people felt upset by what they were writing because it brought up some difficult feelings, but by the third day they were feeling lighter and less burdened by the situations and the feelings. If you feel more burdened, depressed, or upset by day three or especially day four, that's a signal to get some professional help. The purpose of this exercise is not to get bogged down in these memories, it's to acknowledge them, feel them, and begin to move past them.

If at any time you find you cannot forgive yourself to such an extent that you get and stay depressed, you should seek out professional psychological and/or spiritual help. If you decide to do that, find a professional who has had training, or at least has read and understands the approach of Dr. Lawrence LeShan in working with people with cancer. LeShan, author of *Cancer as a Turning Point*, believes that psychological work should be directed toward what "turns you on" and stimulates your vitality, rather than on an analysis of how you got to be the way you are. The only point of addressing the guilt/blame/shame issue is if it is a barrier to your healing work. If it is, get some help to clear it out enough so you can move forward. If not, steam right on ahead!

How can I make my imagery more powerful?

Take the time to relax and focus inside: When you take the time to concentrate on virtually anything you do, whatever you are doing tends to come out better. The same is true of imagery practices. Taking the time to relax, to shift your attention from the outer to the inner world, helps you concentrate better on the imagery and tends to intensify the effects of the imagery.

If I asked you now to make a sandwich, turn on the TV to a show you like, all the while thinking about all the things you need to do in the coming week, it would be difficult for you simultaneously to imagine that you are in a quiet peaceful place with nothing to do. The relaxing effect of the imagery will be diluted compared to the effect you'd experience by stretching out, breathing deeply, relaxing your body, and focusing on what you see, hear, smell, and feel in that special place. Taking the time to focus specifically on your imagery will allow you to learn more about it and experience its positive effects more quickly and intensely than if you just think about it in the midst of everything else you do. So set aside some time, at least once a day, just to focus inside and work with imagery. Taking even more time is almost undoubtedly better, and most studies that have looked at the physiologic effects of imagery have studied people that use it at least twice a day, for about 20 to 30 minutes at a time.

One way to understand the utility of taking the time to relax and focus on your imagery is that it tends to increase what an engineer would call the signal to noise ratio in your thinking. It's like tuning in the radio precisely to a station you want to hear; if you are in between stations, you get static and background noise that makes it both more difficult and less enjoyable to listen to, whereas if you can tune in precisely you hear the beauty of the music with little distraction.

If you are like most modern people, you might be trying to pay attention to several things at once in the course of your average day. Multitasking is a highly rewarded trait in our society, and the ability to do or track several things at once is a hallmark of a highly productive person. Unfortunately, it frequently means that not every item gets your full attention and whatever you are doing suffers.

As you learn to use your mind to help support your healing, it only makes sense that there should be at least *some* time spent where your attention is undivided and solely focused on the business at hand. When you pay full attention, several things happen:

 ✦ You observe more details about the process and are able to perceive things about your illness, its healing, and your mind/body connection that you may have overlooked when it was only one of the many things that get your partial attention.

* The energy in your full attention is necessarily more focused and concentrated than when you are in scanning mode. In some ways it is comparable to the difference between the broad, soft illumination from an incandescent lightbulb and the powerful focused beams of a laser. The lightbulb can illuminate a room, but the laser can cut through steel. To the extent that the energy focused by your attention actually does "work" in the sense of creating physical change in its path, it is likely to be more efficient when it is concentrated.

* In this highly focused state, the images you focus on become more subjectively real, that is, they take up the foreground of your awareness and your body tends to react to them as it would if you were actually in the situations you are imagining. Putting distractions aside and taking some time to focus only on what you imagine seeing, hearing, smelling, and feeling makes the scenario more subjectively real to the lower brain centers that signal the deep autonomic responses of the body. In other words, as you get more immersed in your imagery, the outer world slips away (or at least your awareness of it does) and your body begins to respond more and more as if what you are imagining is really taking place. If you're imagining being in a peaceful place, you'll begin to feel peaceful; if you imagine something sexual, you'll get turned on; if you imagine something exciting or scary, you'll get excited or scared, and if you imagine something healing— what do you think might happen?

* Taking the time to relax and do healing imagery reduces your stress and gives you the experience of doing something active to help yourself. Maintaining stress control is an important part of winning the mind-body game with cancer, and the practice can only help make it better.

* Regular times to relax and focus on healing allows your physiology to balance itself. In deep relaxation, the body goes into a state of enhanced repair and replenishment all by itself. Balancing of physiology is a bonus "side effect" of relaxation practice when you take regular time for healing. While you may be doing other things when you imagine stimulating your immunity, shifting blood flow, and

employing other means of healing, you are also doing it in a state of focused relaxation and awareness that by itself has multiple benefits for your well-being.

Practice regularly: I generally encourage patients to take time at least once each day where they put everything else aside and focus single-mindedly on the aspect of healing that is most important that day—whether it is sorting information, decision making, problem solving, imagery rehearsal, or healing imagery. Take the time to enter a relatively relaxed, quiet state of mind-body awareness and focus on what is most important.

It may be that the time you dedicate to imagery is cumulative in its effects or it may simply indicate that you feel it's worthy of your full attention. Both are probably important and helpful. When you take the time to focus only on healing, it signals to the healing powers that be that healing is of real importance to you—it is high on your priority list, you are serious about it, and you are willing to invest time and energy in it.

Reinforce your healing imagery by thinking of it often: Rachel Naomi Remen, M.D., the author of *Kitchen Table Wisdom* and *My Grandfather's Blessings*, says that she always encourages people to think briefly about healing imagery throughout their day in the same way we normally worry: "We don't sit down for twenty minutes in a meditative posture to worry, do we?" In addition to however many formal sessions you do, think about healing within you often, even for a few seconds. Make everything you do part of your healing—every bite of food, everything you enjoy, every treatment you take. You learned to do this to replace useless worrying a while back, but you can do it for the pleasure of stimulating healing, too, even if you're not worrying.

Pay attention to the images that spontaneously form when you focus on healing: When you relax and pay attention to your imagery, you make room for other information that may be unconscious to come to the fore. This information can be important if not crucial to helping you deal with your cancer experience. This aspect of imagery can be facilitated by including your Inner Healer in your healing process. Have a visit with it periodically to see if there's anything else that you might include in your healing efforts.

Use multiple views of your healing: Should your healing imagery focus on the physiologic process of healing or on the ultimate outcome? Is it better if your imagery is anatomically and physiologically accurate, or is it more powerful if it's symbolic? The research doesn't yet tell us. A case can be made for either side of these issues, but it costs nothing more to utilize them all and cover all the bases.

I encourage you to consider including four areas in your healing imagery:

1. Imagery that represents or symbolizes the physical healing you desire, however you imagine it. Include here images that represent your immune or cancer defense responses, and the actions of any therapies you are employing, whether conventionally medical or alternative. Imagine your treatments working perfectly—just as they would work if it were totally up to you. Imagine any cancer cells or tumor tissue being walled off, destroyed, and eliminated from your body—whether by force fields, chemical poisons and aggressive swarming immune cells, or by any other mechanism.

2. Imagine the outcome you desire in a "bigger picture" format—we sometimes call this *future pacing*. Imagine yourself in the future, as far as you'd like to imagine yourself living, feeling well, thriving, and doing what you love to do with whomever you love to do it. This is the place to imagine yourself at future events that are important to you—weddings, graduations, births, and other landmark events. Imagine these happening in the present and let yourself get into them as completely as you can, seeing what you see, hearing what you hear, feeling what you feel. Imagine a calendar with the date on it as you do this, and enjoy it as much as possible.

3. A variation of the last focus is useful if you have felt discouraged or scared by any of your doctor's predictions or reactions. Include as

one of your desired outcomes being with your doctor in his or her office, with a calendar on the wall with a date circled, with you, the doctor, and anyone else who accompanies you feeling great, happy, all celebrating the good news the doctor has just given you—that there is no progression or no cancer at all. Imagine your doctor's response—from puzzlement to excitement, and notice any good feelings you have about overcoming their initial predictions.

4. If your belief system includes a spiritual aspect, pray or ask for help from the creator who looks over you, guides you, and protects you, and let yourself know that with this help you are fully capable of meeting whatever challenge or opportunity may come your way in life. If spirituality is not a part of your life, let yourself know that by yourself, and with the support of others you may choose to include, you are fully capable of meeting whatever challenge or opportunity may come your way in life.

Use multiple senses in your imagery: Let me clarify a common misconception about imagery—it's not all visual. Humans are primarily visual animals, and for most of us, vision is our dominant sense. When we imagine things, we think of picturing things in our mind's eye. Studies have found that about 85 percent of people do visualize, but imagery, being a type of sensory-based thinking, also utilizes other senses—hearing, smell, touch, even taste. Some people do not visualize at all, but almost everyone can imagine—and that's what is important.

Sometimes people are inhibited because they think they are not good visualizers, but we all imagine one way or another. Take some time to notice how you imagine things and let yourself accept that for now. There's no evidence I'm aware of to say that visualization works better than any other type of imagining. When people tell me they can't visualize, I often ask them a simple question: "Can you imagine a friendly dragon?" Most people say, "Sure," and then I ask them to describe their dragon. Without closing their eyes, doing any relaxation, or going into a trance state they usually say something like, "Well, it's green." I ask what color its eyes are and they say, "Yellow."

I ask what it's doing and they say, "Oh, it's just sitting there with some smoke coming out of its nostrils."

How do *you* imagine a friendly dragon? What does your dragon look like? What color is it? What's it doing? How close or far away from you is it? Would you like to touch it to see what it feels like? What's that like? Does it smell or have an odor? How do you feel toward it?

Do you actually *see* this dragon in your mind, or do you imagine it some other way? Notice how you imagine this and accept that your way of imagining is just as good as any other.

When you do healing imagery you will be encouraged to pay attention to all of your senses. Some people have sensations when they imagine certain things, while others don't. Some imagine smells, for example; others don't, which is fine. I am going to strongly and repetitively encourage you to accept the way you naturally imagine things, especially at the beginning. As you learn more about working with imagery, you may find that the way you imagine things changes and you can refine what you are doing if that feels important to you.

Make your imagery congruent with your treatment choices: While many people imagine that healing with cancer involves a battle or fight, I've known some people who have imagined instead that their cancer was healed by cells coming back into alignment with the body's normal cells. Some of these people have imagined light and love as the most powerful healing agent, which it may well be. On occasion they have had some difficulty with imagery because their imagery is of healing through love while they are irradiating or poisoning cancer cells. I think you have to find some way of resolving this discrepancy—if you are killing cancer cells, then kill cancer cells.

Greg is a 44-year-old man who fought a tough but successful battle with lung cancer. A peaceful sort by nature, he felt badly about using aggressive imagery for healing. One day he went to visit our local Museum of Natural History and saw a tableau that showed an Eskimo hunter standing over the body of a seal he had just killed. Greg learned that the hunter, like most of those from native cultures, prayed to the soul of any creature he killed, thanking it for bringing its life-sustaining nourishment. Greg understood that he could kill cancer cells, while "thanking" them for bringing his awareness to his health in a new way, and imagining that the new cells that took their place were welcomed into place with love and healing energy.

Make sure your imagery is congruent with your treatments—whether they be medical, surgical, nutritional, or other—otherwise you can be sure you are simply indulging in fantasy and not using your intention coherently.

How can I make my imagery more tangible?

For some people, imagery is too intangible to work with. If this applies to you, try making it more tangible by writing and drawing about what these images would be like. What do you imagine healing would look like if you could witness it in your body? What will you be like if you fully recover? What will you be doing? What will be different, if anything, about you? What will you treasure and attend to even more?

You can also use a Gestalt therapy technique in which you imagine that your Inner Advisor or Healer is sitting in a chair across from you. Say what you'd like to say to it, then get up and exchange places, physically. Sitting in the other chair, let yourself speak as your advisor or healer and answer the self you imagine is still sitting in the first chair. Keep switching chairs, and every time you switch, take a little time to consider what you have just heard. Respond honestly and with caring each time from the appropriate perspective. You can also use this technique to explore any other "image" or part of you that you'd like to know more about, perhaps the part of you that objects to imagining.

Another way to strengthen the tangibility and power of imagination is by externalizing your imagery. Even if you are comfortable with imagery, you may also want to include some of these external measures to augment it.

Consider creating a special place for healing work in your home, your garden, or anywhere else there is room to create what could be called a sacred space. This could be an altar, a corner of a room, or anywhere you want to consecrate, perhaps by saying a prayer or affirmation, or using a ritual like burning sage or a candle. If you don't have such an external space, remember that you can create such a space internally when you go to your healing place inside. Add anything to it that makes it more beautiful, more powerful, and more healing for you, and keep adding things as you learn more about your relationship to healing.

You may want to draw, paint, or sculpt a place of healing, a symbol of healing, or even an Inner Advisor or Healer. You could make immune cells out of clay and a model of them eating cancer cells. Don't worry about the artistic quality; just let it be something that makes it more tangible for you. You can share your creations with others if you like, but you don't have to. If you find yourself spending more time and energy criticizing your poor art or imagery skills than creating images of healing, you are going in an unproductive direction. Drop the self-criticism and concentrate on what you imagine is healing.

I'm a big fan of the Mel Brooks school of psychotherapy. You may remember his "2000-year-old man" who claimed to have experienced almost everything over his long lifetime. He claimed to have cured an old woman that even founders of psychotherapy Freud, Jung, and Adler couldn't cure. She compulsively ripped paper all day long. He said he cured her in one session. "That's amazing! How did you do that?" asked Carl Reiner, his straight man. "I told her, *Stop ripping paper! What are you doing, ripping paper all day long? Stop it!*" So, if you find yourself wallowing in self-criticism, stop it! If you can't get over it, then work with a qualified imagery guide or psychotherapist to help you get over the hump. It's just not a good use of your mind.

Another useful technique for people who have trouble with imagery is to create affirmations of their healing. An affirmation is a statement usually beginning with the phrase "I am . . ." or "I can . . ." or "I will . . ."—a phrase that you can repeat to yourself frequently to calm, stimulate, or remind yourself about what you want to keep in focus. Thus a simple affirmation like "I am an incredible self-healer" or "I can get better from this" or "I will do whatever I can to help my healing" can be a handy thought to go to, especially if your fears come up, as we discussed in chapter 2. This way, even if you can't do healing imagery, you can energize your intention to heal.

If you are already comfortable with imagery, verbal affirmations can add another dimension to your self-suggestions for healing. Say you are too tired to focus well on imagery—it's easy to do affirmations, which provide a touchstone or reminder of your intention. Some people create affirmations that they mentally repeat as a mantra or chant.

You might also consider singing, humming, or making a sound that reminds you of your healing power. There may be a phrase from a song that catches you or comes to mind that speaks of healing, peace, courage, or whatever you want to cultivate in yourself. It could just be a sound. The reason cats heal so quickly may have to do with their purring, according to some emerging evidence. It may be that the regular vibration helps to organize the tissues that are healing.

How do you imagine your healing sound? Take some time in a quiet (and private) place and experiment making tones and sounds—see what brings energy to different parts of your body, and notice if any of it feels especially calming or healing to you. Traditional Tibetan medicine has used toning as a means of healing for thousands of years, and a prominent progressive oncologist, Mitchell Gaynor, uses Tibetan bells along with imagery to augment the self-healing process in his patients.[2]

You may also want to experiment with music as a background for your imagery. Music often amplifies imagery and has a close connection with it. In the field called Guided Imagery in Music, pioneered by psychologist Helen Bonny, trained therapists use special selections of music to help people access certain emotions. Different emotions tend to evoke different images. Some music is soothing and relaxing, some is ethereal and inspirational, while other pieces are warlike and heroic. Music encourages imagery that is congruent with the moods it evokes. Choose music that helps to create the feelings and qualities you need to appropriately fuel the imagery you intend to do. I like using nature sounds or the music of Stephen Halpern, who has been called the "Mozart of the New Age." His music, tonal and evocative, is perfect for relaxation and imagery.

Your sense of smell can be highly evocative in imagery, and the evolving science of aromatherapy attempts to utilize this connection. Perhaps because the olfactory nerve (the nerve you smell with) goes directly back into the limbic, or emotional, brain, smell can be a powerful activator of emotions and of imagery. You might investigate the aromatherapy section of your health food store to see what effects different aromas have on your mood and imagery. If you find aromas that feel especially healing, and use them along with your healing imagery, you may soon be able to use the aroma to trigger the healing responses you create in your body.

This, of course, is the classical use of a process called conditioning, discovered by the famous Russian scientist Ivan Pavlov in the early part of the twentieth century. Pavlov found that if he rang a bell whenever he put food out for his dogs, his dogs would soon begin to salivate when they heard the bell ring, whether food was there or not.

What's important about this for you? Let's say that you activate your immune and healing responses whenever you do healing imagery, and each time you do this you simultaneously do something else—like touching your thumb and index finger together, touching a stone or jewel you associate with healing, saying an affirmation, or smelling an aromatherapy oil. The healing responses will get conditioned to whatever else you do and give you an easy way to enhance your healing.

One of the seminal experiments that helped legitimize the science of psychoneuroimmunology took advantage of this conditioning effect. Robert Ader and his colleagues at the University of Rochester had mice drink water that was laced with saccharine and a drug that suppressed the immune system. Once the mice were conditioned to this, they were given simple saccharine water, without any drug, and were found to suppress their own immune systems. Pairing your healing imagery or rituals with simple movements, aromas, or affirmations makes a lot of sense; it can give you a way to reinforce the healing you are doing in simple, time-efficient ways.

Another powerful way to express and augment your imagery is to combine it with movement. Making physical movements gets the body involved and externalizes the imagery so it becomes more tangible to you. Renowned dancer Anna Halprin has evolved a method for this, which she calls "psychokinetic visualization." If this is of interest to you, her remarkable book, *Dance as a Self-Healing Art*, is a must-read.

If you utilize some or all of these external aids, you may want to develop a healing ceremony or ritual that strengthens your connection to the healing process. Some people create private rituals only for themselves, while others invite friends, family, and healing helpers to the ritual. It may be a traditional one, like a Native American sweat lodge, or one of your own creation. The important thing is that it contain elements that are genuinely meaningful to you. *Rituals of Healing* by Jeanne Achterberg, Leslie Kolkmeier, and Barbara Dossey is a wonderful resource to learn more about creating healing rituals and integrating them into your imagery.

Whatever you do to externally augment, represent, or amplify your imagery, don't confuse the external aspects with the healing. Let the rituals affect you: draw from their power, take it inside, and imagine that it is doing exactly what you want it to do.

What if I have trouble imagining healing at all?

If you are still having trouble with imagery, there are two possibilities to consider. The first is that you may be discounting your imagery because you feel it's "not good enough." Usually, this is part of a larger "not good enough" thinking pattern. If this describes you, what are you comparing your imagery to? How do you know that your way is "not good enough"? The stories I share with you in this book come from people who have vivid images as well as those who just accept the thoughts that come to them when they ask for images. Please do the same for yourself.

The second possibility is that you have some unconscious concern about imagining healing. Perhaps a part of you feels that if it imagines healing and it works, you are somehow at fault for your disease. Perhaps a part of you feels that it smacks of mysticism or is vaguely heretical. Or there could be a part that feels if you really put your heart into imagining healing and it doesn't work you will be too devastated to go on. These are hard concerns to let yourself become aware of because they contradict what you are trying to do. If they are present, though, it's important to find a way to work with these issues and move toward reaching your healing goals.

You can use the imagery dialogue approach to explore this issue. Relax and go inside to your place of healing, ask your Inner Healer to be there with you, then ask if there is any part of you that has any concern or objection to imagining the healing process. If you get a sense there is, you can invite an image of that part of you to appear in your special healing place so you can find out its concerns. Take some time to get to know the image, and let it express its concerns or fears. Don't judge it or try to change it before thoroughly understanding what its concerns are. Then, see if you can find a way to attend to its concerns while still helping yourself move toward healing. Ask the part itself and your Inner Healer to help you imagine how this could happen.

A brief example may serve to show how this can be achieved. Grace was a sixty-year-old woman with metastatic melanoma who came to me for help with her healing imagery. She was having difficulty imagining her immune system vigorously fighting her tumor. Her imagery consisted of a few relatively inert immune cells sitting on her image of the tumor, which she described as a "blob." Many suggestions and interventions by me failed to increase the activity, until I asked her to allow an image to form for anything standing in the way of her imagining her healing. Grace then saw herself standing at the edge of a large chasm, her husband and grown children on the other side. They were waving for her to come across the chasm. She began to cry at this image, the first evidence I had seen of emotion in our half-dozen sessions.

I asked about her tears and she told me that the one regret she had was that her family was emotionally distant and estranged from each other and she hadn't been able to change that. I asked her what she wanted to do in her imagery and she said she needed to build a bridge to reach them. She then built an imaginary bridge and imagined walking across into the welcoming arms of her embracing family.

When we discussed this experience, I asked her if there was anything she wanted to do differently in her outer life as a result of what she had imagined. She decided to ask her family to meet together with a family therapist, something they had never done. After a short series of deeply moving sessions the family banded together in a way it never had before. Subsequently Grace's healing imagery became vigorous and active, as did her participation in other aspects of her treatment, including nutrition, exercise, and an experimental clinical trial of a medical treatment.

Grace's willingness to explore whatever was in the way of doing more vigorous healing imagery allowed her to identify and resolve an emotional barrier that she never logically connected to this process. The benefits her family experienced as a result of this insight and action allowed her to fight much more enthusiastically for her health.

What we often call resistance, then, is not necessarily a bad thing. Consider that there may be a legitimate reason holding you back and make an honest effort to let it come to mind—then you can work toward finding a way to address your concern and move forward wholeheartedly.

Another way to explore this issue is to have a talk with your Inner Advisor or Healer and ask for some help in resolving it.

How can I imagine healing when my tests show the cancer is still there?

The paradox of guided imagery and most mind-body approaches that involve suggestion could be described as "fake it till you make it." You set the goal and direction in which you want to move with an image. Some people think that once they've imagined something happening, it has happened at some level of reality. This may or may not be so, but with this issue we are concerned with the physical level of reality, your cancer. It is not likely to go up in a ball of smoke the first time you imagine that happening.

If you're trying to hit a bull's-eye with a dart, you have a much better chance of hitting it if you keep your eye on the target. It doesn't guarantee that you'll hit it, but if you keep trying and keep intending to hit the target, and keep throwing darts, your nervous and musculoskeletal systems will do their best to hit that bull's-eye, and over time you will throw more darts closer to the center and hit more bull's-eyes than before. That's the way we are made. Pick a target that means something to you and stay focused on it and you will mobilize all the resources you have to hit that target. The same principle applies to healing.

Patience and perseverance go a long way here. The *I Ching*, the ancient Chinese book of wisdom, says that though the wind may be invisible and much less solid than the land, it can shape the land when it persistently blows in the same direction.

*What aspects of physical healing
can imagery potentially influence?*

IMMUNITY

The most common imagery that people do to imagine physical healing is the attack on cancer cells or tumors by immune defenders in one guise or another. In their early research on imagery and cancer, the Simontons predicted that this process could boost immune cell function against cancer long before the results could be measured, and numerous studies have now shown this to be true. Imagining that your immune system, or cancer defense system, actively removes any cancer cells or tissue from your body is usually an important part of imagery programs for healing cancer. But there are other physical elements of the body's ability to protect and defend that you might also focus on in your healing imagery.

BLOOD FLOW

An important physiologic function that has a great deal to do with healing is blood flow. A lot of current medical research focuses on ways to stop cancer from creating its own blood supply. Some cancers have the ability to stimulate production of new blood vessels to feed their growing demands (a process called angiogenesis) and shutting off that blood supply would deprive the tumor of its source of nourishment. Could we potentially do that with our minds?

There is good reason to believe that it could happen. Extensive research demonstrates that people using biofeedback devices to monitor temperature are able to warm or cool their extremities by altering blood flow. This can be very specific. It has even been shown that people can create large temperature differences between two points on the back of one hand if they get feedback that tells them what they are doing. Even more startling is the finding, discussed later in chapter 7 on surgical preparation, that ordinary people, without any biofeedback of any kind, are able to shunt blood flow away from the site of surgery simply by being told they can. They reduced their surgical blood loss by nearly half, which indicates that we may have a much greater ability to control our blood flow than we ever thought. Why not include it in your intentional imaging of healing?

Studies investigating hypnosis and warts have used suggestions that include the idea that the wart is fed blood through a single capillary that enters from the bottom, and that the blood supply can be cut off by shutting the valve that controls the flow of the blood—like a valve shuts off your water supply to a sink or toilet. Imagining shutting off the blood supply to tumors, or that they are surrounded by some sort of encapsulation that isolates them from blood and nutrients and prevents them from eliminating their waste products, is a common imagery my patients use. They imagine such tumors starving, shriveling, and dissolving in their own waste products, and the debris being cleaned up by an efficient immune system. Of course, your own image is the best, but use these common ones if a powerful image doesn't come to mind.

If you wanted to make the best use of this potential healing, you might imagine opening such a valve when you receive chemotherapy so that the chemotherapy medication permeates the tumor, then imagine closing the valve to let the tumor soak in the poison. You might imagine opening the valve after five days and imagine the dead cells and debris being washed away and leaving your body through your stools, urine, breath, and sweat. Then you may imagine an ebullient, aggressive swarm of immune cells devouring the rest of the tumor if any were left, and once that was done, turning off the valve again so that any tumor remnant received no nourishment or blood supply at all.

ONCOGENES

A third mechanism of cancer formation involves what is known as oncogenes, genes that can either induce or inhibit the formation of cancer cells. Oncogenes are regulatory genes, which means they turn on and off—most of the time we don't know why, but it is interesting to note that they can be turned off.

There is a lot of emphasis on the genetic predisposition to cancer these days and much hope that genetic alteration will one day be helpful to people with cancer. But the fact is that most people with genetic traits that make them more likely to get cancer still don't actually get the disease. For example, the BRCA 1 and 2 genes that predispose some Ashkenazi Jewish women to breast and ovarian cancers increase the likelihood by ten to thirty times that they will develop one of these cancers. But the majority of women with one of those genes still do not develop cancer—so the gene is not the only factor. This is true of the vast majority of genetically influenced cancers.

What other factors are believed to influence whether the cancer gene is activated and is able to create an actual cancer? Environmental influences are suspect—from radiation damage due to X rays or ambient radiation, to tumor-promoting or tumor-inhibiting nutrient factors, to chemical changes that accompany prolonged or severe stress. We don't know all the factors yet. But if you are going to use your mind to try to influence the course of your cancer, why not imagine exactly what you want to have happen, and let the chips (or genes) fall where they may? Imagine you can turn the genetic switch to "off." Let your unconscious, your spirit, your body know what you want. And get out of the way.

Following is a guided imagery process that can allow you to revisit, update, and refine your healing imagery. It will give you opportunities to imagine images discussed in this chapter and see if other things you've learned or experienced in your cancer treatment to date can now be included. There are many ways to talk about healing, and many ways to imagine it. Notice how you imagine healing now.

Your All-Inclusive Healing Imagery

Take a comfortable position and let yourself begin to relax in your own way . . . let your breathing get a little deeper and fuller . . . but still comfortable . . . with every breath in, notice that you bring in fresh air, fresh oxygen, fresh energy that fuels your body . . . and with every breath out, imagine that you can release a bit of tension . . . a bit of discomfort . . . a bit of worry . . . and let that deeper breathing and the thoughts you have of fresh energy in and tension and worry out be an invitation to your body and mind to begin to relax . . . to begin to shift gears . . . and let it be an easy and natural movement . . . without having to force anything . . . without having to make anything happen right

now . . . just letting it happen . . . just breathing and relaxing . . . breathing and energizing. . . .

Come back to taking a few deeper breaths whenever you feel like relaxing even more deeply . . . but for now, let your breathing take its own natural rate and its own natural rhythm . . . and simply let the gentle movement of your body as it breathes allow you to relax naturally and comfortably . . . almost without having to try. . . .

And noticing how your right foot feels right now . . . and how your left foot feels . . . and noticing that just before you probably weren't aware of your feet at all . . . but now that you turn your attention to them, you can notice them and how they feel . . . and notice the intelligence that is there in your feet . . . and notice what happens when you silently invite your feet to relax . . . and become soft and at ease . . . and in the same way noticing the intelligence in your legs and releasing your legs . . . and letting the intelligence in your legs respond in their own way . . . and noticing any release and relaxation that happens . . . without having to make any effort at all . . . just softening and releasing . . . and letting it be a comfortable and very pleasant experience. . . .

And you can relax even more deeply and comfortably if you want to . . . by continuing to notice the intelligence in different parts of your body and inviting them to soften and relax . . . and noticing how they relax . . . and you are in control of your relaxation and only relax as deeply as is comfortable for you . . . and if you ever need to return your awareness to the outer world you can do that by opening your eyes and looking around and coming fully alert . . . and if you need to respond to anything there you can do that . . . and knowing that you can do this if you need to . . . you can relax again and return your attention to the inner world of your imagination. . . .

Inviting the intelligence of your low back, pelvis, and hips to release and relax . . . and your abdomen and midsection . . . and your chest and rib cage . . . without effort or struggle . . . just letting go but staying aware as you do. . . .

Inviting the intelligence in your back and spine to soften and release . . . in your low back . . . mid-back . . . between and across your shoulder blades . . . and across your neck and shoulders . . . the intelligence in your arms . . . and elbows . . . and forearms . . . through your wrists and hands . . . and the palms of the hands . . . the fingers . . . and thumbs. . . .

Noticing the intelligence in your face and jaws and inviting them to relax . . . to become soft and at ease . . . and your scalp and forehead . . . and your eyes . . . even your tongue can be at ease. . . .

And as you relax, let your attention shift from your usual outer world to what we can call your inner world . . . the world inside that only you can see, hear, smell, and feel . . . the world where your memories, your dreams, your feelings, your plans all reside . . . a world that you can learn to connect with . . . that can help you in many ways on your journey. . . .

And imagine that you find inside a very special place . . . a very beautiful place where you feel comfortable and relaxed, yet very aware . . . this may be a place that you have actually visited at some time in your life . . . in the outer world or even in this inner world . . . or it may be a place that you've seen somewhere . . . or it may be a brand-new place that you haven't visited before . . . and none of that matters as long as it is a very beautiful place, a place that invites you and feels good to be in . . . a place that feels safe and healing for you. . . .

And let yourself take some time to explore this place . . . and notice what you imagine seeing there . . . all the things you

see . . . and how you see them . . . don't worry at all about how
you imagine this place as long as it is beautiful to you and feels
safe and healing . . . and notice if there are any sounds you imagine hearing . . . or if it is simply very quiet in your healing
place . . . notice if there is a fragrance or aroma that you imagine
there or a special quality of the air . . . there may or may not be,
and it's perfectly all right however you imagine this place of healing . . . it may change over time as you explore it, or it may stay
the same . . . it doesn't matter at this point . . . just let yourself
explore a little more. . . .

Can you tell what time of day it is . . . or what time of year it
is? . . . and what the temperature is like? . . . how you are
dressed? . . . take some time to find a place where you feel safe
and let yourself get comfortable there . . . and just notice how it
feels to imagine yourself there . . . and if your mind wanders from
time to time, just take another deep breath or two and gently
return your attention to this beautiful and healing place . . . just
for now . . . without feeling the need to go anywhere else right
now . . . or do anything else . . . just for now. . . .

And as you relax in this special place of healing, let an image
come to mind that can now symbolize the healing that is already
going on within you . . . and the strength and abilities of the healing systems built into your body . . . let an image come that represents this to you—it may come in any form . . . it may be the
same image that you have had before, or it could be a new
image . . . notice what comes to mind as you invite an image for
healing . . . how would you imagine yourself full of healing
energy and activity and feeling whole, healthy, and strong? . . . let
yourself begin to imagine yourself that way now . . . and don't
worry at all about whether the image you have now is the best
image or the strongest image . . . you may well come up with
many images of your healing as you work through this
process . . . and may change your imagery many times to better

fit your understanding of the process . . . but for now, let this image you have stand for the healing your body, mind, and spirit can do . . . and imagine it happening now in you . . . and imagine it being as strong and powerful and effective as you possibly can . . . if you need more power, imagine you can connect to people and things you love . . . and to whatever source of life and energy you imagine put you here in the first place . . . and imagine that those provide powerful sources of healing energy that you can direct throughout your body, mind, and spirit to heal what needs to be healed . . . to eliminate what needs to be eliminated . . . and to repair what needs to be repaired. . . .

Imagine that any treatments you are taking are working beautifully . . . and that you can shut off any blood supply to any remaining tumor . . . and that your immune defense systems completely and thoroughly eradicate any remaining abnormal cells . . . and that they are excreted from your body whenever it eliminates. . . .

And imagine that your spirit and brain can turn off any genes that need to be turned off so that there are no further instructions for any abnormal cells and any remaining cells in the body divide and grow healthy and cooperatively. . . .

Take a few minutes now and imagine this happening in your own way and let whatever way you imagine this happening to be just fine for now . . . your unconscious mind understands what your conscious mind is telling it . . . it understands that your intention is to activate and stimulate all the healing capabilities it has . . . and it knows just how to respond, however you imagine this healing. . . .

(Pause for 15 seconds)

And imagine too yourself in the future . . . doing the things you love to do . . . with whomever you love to do them with . . . and feeling healthy and vital and enjoying it . . . and imagine yourself enjoying any special events or dates that you would like to attend in the future . . . and imagine that you are there now . . . and see the date on a calendar that you can imagine . . . and there may be more than one. . . .

Imagine yourself in your doctor's office in the future and imagine the dates on a calendar on the wall . . . it may be one with pages that fly off as they do in old-time movies . . . see you and your doctor happy and pleased with the outcome of your latest tests . . . feeling good about them . . . and about how you are. . . .

Let an image come to mind that can encapsulate or represent this whole healing process for you . . . a particular image or "film clip" of imagery that can stand for this whole process . . . and anytime you find yourself worrying about cancer or how it will affect you, let yourself stay with that for as long as it spurs you to think creatively about how you can resolve that concern . . . and as soon as you become aware that your fears and worries are simply fears or worries, acknowledge them . . . and imagine that you can cancel the fear or worry . . . imagine having a big red circle with a slash through it on a rubber stamp and stamp that fear out . . . and touch your thumbs to your fingers to reconnect you with your focus on healing . . . and replace worry with your current image of healing . . . and any word or phrase that also affirms it for you . . . and let yourself sit with that imagery of healing for a few moments more, noticing how it feels to imagine that happening in you now . . . and knowing that this can get even more powerful as you learn to use your imagination even better for healing. . . .

And you can let the images and feelings of healing stay with you as long as you like and even bring them back with you when you decide to return your attention to the outer world. . . .

And taking all the time you need. . . .

(Pause for 20 seconds)

And when you are ready to return your attention to the outer world, silently express any appreciation you might have for having a special healing place within you . . . and for being able to use your imagination in this way . . . and for the healing capabilities that have been built into you by nature . . . and when you are ready, allow all the images to fade and go back within . . . knowing that healing continues to happen within you at all times . . . and gently bring your attention back to the room around you and the current time and place . . . and bring back with you anything that seems important or interesting to bring back, including any feelings of comfort, relaxation, or healing . . . and when you are all the way back, gently stretch and open your eyes. . . .

And take a few minutes to write or draw about your experience.

Debriefing Your Experience

What was this experience like for you? Was your healing imagery different in any way from before, or the same? If you haven't already, consider drawing, painting, or modeling your healing imagery now. Don't worry about artistic merit—this is for you, to help you make it more tangible and real.

What seems especially important or interesting to you about your healing imagery now?

What questions do you have about your healing imagery?

What might your Inner Healer say about these questions? Consider a visit with your Inner Healer to address them.

Summary

✦ Humans are organized so that we try to achieve goals we set.

✦ Healing imagery is a type of goal-setting that can restore a sense of psychological control, stimulate physiologic responses in the body, prime your unconscious mind to detect and become aware of healing opportunities, and mobilize the mystery to come to your aid.

✦ Imagining healing can take many forms, but the best images are *your* images.

✦ Practicing your imagery regularly, using more senses, and using ritual, conditioning cues, and movement can amplify the effects of healing imagery.

✦ Make your healing imagery congruent with your treatment choices, that is, if you are trying to kill cancer cells with chemotherapy or radiation, imagine those treatments working perfectly.

✦ An extended healing imagery process allows you to refine and update your healing imagery to include all you've learned and experienced.

6

Making Good Decisions

Whatever you can do or dream you can, begin it.
Boldness has genius, power, and magic in it.
—Johann Wolfgang von Goethe

When you are diagnosed with cancer, you will be asked to make important decisions about your treatment that you may feel ill-prepared to make. Sometimes the facts point to relatively straightforward treatment decisions, although even these may not be easy to make since they involve choosing discomfort or becoming temporarily ill. At other times, the decisions may be so difficult that even experts who have studied these matters for years will have disagreements and conflicted opinions.

The one decision that only you can make is the decision to commit to doing whatever will help you beat the disease. Dick Block, founder of H&R Block, who survived an advanced case of lung cancer, writes passionately, in his book *Fighting Cancer*:

> You must, on your own, make the commitment that you will do everything in your power to fight your disease. No exceptions. Nothing halfway. Nothing for the sake of ease or convenience. Everything! Nothing short of it. When you have done this, you have accomplished the most difficult thing you will have to accomplish throughout your entire treatment.

It may seem strange to think that there would be any trouble making that decision, but cancer treatment can be difficult and long. It requires courage and the willingness to suffer treatments that can sometimes make you feel tired and ill. It can be expensive and wearing on you and your family. But the people I've seen who have beaten serious cancers have fought the cancer all the way, mobilizing themselves and all their resources, finding the right doctors and other professionals, changing their lifestyles, using everything they think will help them and using their minds powerfully and well.

Once you've committed yourself, you will then need to decide what treatments are the best for you. You might think that making treatment decisions would be a primarily rational process, involving clarification of the decision to be made; gathering the information necessary in order to make an informed decision; evaluating the risk/benefit ratio and consequences of the decisions; and choosing the best one for you.

However, a number of confounding factors will come into play that interfere with or compete with pure rationality. It's useful to familiarize yourself with them so you can make the best decision for you.

First, the guidelines that are supposed to help you make these decisions may not be clear. You will be choosing between treatments (or no treatment) but what are you really choosing? Most people, and most oncologists, assume that a patient will choose conventional treatment because he or she is so uncomfortable "doing nothing." (Although a patient choosing alternative treatments or doing mind-body work is not "doing nothing.") Yet many commonly accepted cancer treatment protocols do not even have survival as their goal—the research may instead report on other end-points, such as remission or improved quality of life. While these outcomes are certainly not without value, you should know what the oncologist feels he or she can reasonably offer you with each treatment offered. It may change your decision.

Consider asking these questions of each oncologist you interview: Is there a likelihood, or even a chance of cure with this treatment? Do more people survive if they take this treatment? If so, by how much, and what difference is there, percentage-wise? Medically, if a treatment offers any increased survival at all, even if it's a few percentage points, we have a tendency to prescribe it, even if it has severe side effects. But a few possible percentage points may or may not be worth suffering for—that's for you to decide.

What's the best outcome your oncologist has ever seen or heard of with this treatment? What are the downsides of treatment? How often do these adverse effects occur? Are these effects permanent or temporary? Are they treatable? Would the doctors have this treatment themselves if they were in the same position? Would the doctor recommend it to a close family member?

When you interview physicians, ask them about the issues that are important to you. For example, some questions you could ask to see how comfortable your physician is with complementary medical approaches are:

What is your experience with people combining medical treatment with nutritional and mind-body treatment?

Do you think that anything I do can help influence the outcome of my treatment?

Will you be willing to work with me to sort out complementary ways to approach my cancer if I choose to explore them?

Asking questions that are important to you helps identify the physicians in whom you can place your confidence. Ideally, you want a doctor with expertise in treating your illness who answers your questions with thoughtfulness and sensitivity. Ideally, you can find expertise, caring, and good communication in one doctor, but if you can't, think about putting together a team that provides all three qualities. Sometimes a team includes an oncologist with the required expertise along with another oncologist or physician who has the communication and caring skills desired. Use both as appropriate.

A dilemma can present itself if you have to choose between a treatment path and a practitioner. At some point, you're going to have to trust somebody, conventional or unconventional. For this reason, in the absence of compelling data I will never steer a patient away from treatments that a trusted oncologist or doctor has suggested. The effect of the trust is too powerful to do without when we don't have a better solution—and we don't know yet whether it's the trust in the "better" solution or the solution itself that has the most power.

Placebo research shows that the effect of positive expectations tends to occur when any of three conditions are met: (1) the patient believes in the doctor; (2) the patient believes in the treatment; and (3) the doctor believes in the treatment. David Bresler, co-director of the Academy for Guided Imagery, insightfully adds, "There's a fourth element that hasn't been studied—the effect of the doctor believing in the healing potential of the patient."

Ask your doctors to treat you as an intelligent, motivated, self-healing dynamo. Ask them if they will support your efforts to heal, as well as treat your disease and help you sort the wheat from the chaff in selecting treatments.

The decisions that are easiest are those that have compelling data to support them and have the best benefit-to-risk ratio. In some situations, we can point to treatments and say that a large majority (or even large number) of people who follow that path are cured, or survive longer, or benefit in other ways, with the side effects temporary, acceptable, or treatable.

In other situations where the data clearly show that medical treatments are not likely to be beneficial many people elect to have them anyway, and doctors agree to prescribe them because we all tend to be insecure without treatment. These situations are those where seeking alternative treatment makes the most sense. Choosing a treatment with little solid evidence of effectiveness but little risk makes sense when compared to a treatment with data showing little effectiveness with significant toxicity.

The most difficult situations arise when there is no consensus on treatment, when the data are conflicting, or where the treatments have some effectiveness but are difficult to tolerate and carry significant risk. This is when utilizing the tools of good decision making is crucial, and when intuition and listening within come more strongly into play.

Decision-Making Tools

Good decisions are based on good information, so knowing how to obtain and evaluate the information you need is crucial. In the not-too-distant past, it was difficult for a patient to get information about medical conditions, especially cancer. The diagnosis of cancer might even be withheld from patients in order to spare them suffering and despair, although this has not been the case for a good forty years in the United States. Now, in addition to what your doctors tell you, there are support and advocacy groups for most types of cancer, medical libraries that are made for patients seeking information, services that will search the world medical literature for you, and a great deal of information you can directly access on the World Wide Web.

Your survival and well-being may depend on your information-gathering and assessment skills. Five years ago, a good friend of mine was found to have cancer in his bladder, and the standard treatment at the time was to have the bladder removed. While it can be life-saving, this is also a difficult, disfiguring, and even disabling treatment. Several leading urologists in the San Francisco Bay area concurred in this recommendation, however.

My friend comes from a family where there's been a lot of cancer, and he's an information technology specialist. As soon as he got out of the hospital he was on the Internet. Within an hour or two, he found a Harvard urologist whose research indicated bladder cancer at his stage could be treated successfully 85 percent of the time—without surgery. The treatment option consisted of chemotherapy instilled into the bladder along with radiation. Following his Internet leads, my friend got this doctor's home telephone number, reached him on a Saturday, and had a lengthy conversation with him about his research protocol.

The doctor sent him his research and my friend reviewed it with the urologist he liked the best, his medical oncologist, and several other doctor friends. The local urologist agreed to follow this protocol with guidance from the Harvard researcher. More than five years later, my friend has his bladder and is cancer-free.

My friend didn't rely on just this treatment, however. He went beyond his already remarkable feat of gathering information and self-assertion to get the *best* treatment. He researched and utilized a wide variety of nutritional, herbal, and psychospiritual support. A longtime meditator and seeker on spiritual paths, he developed a simple visualization and self-message/mantra that "healthy cells grow all by themselves." He joined support groups and actively worked on his attitude and lifestyle. Much of his journey is detailed on his website, at www.yellowstream.com, and is well worth reviewing as an example of not necessarily settling for local expert opinion.

Good information can save your life, or at least your bladder or other bodily functions. That's why it's usually worth taking a little time to carefully check your options. It's common to panic when you hear you have cancer, and you may just feel that you want to get it out of your body as fast as possible. But cancer is most often not an emergency—there is usually some time to gather and sort information before making treatment decisions. How much time? That depends on several factors: the type, location, and stage of the cancer, and how much time you need.

A man in his sixties or seventies with an early nonaggressive prostate cancer could take months to make a decision and probably not increase his risk significantly, whereas a young person with a high-grade lymphoma might need to make a decision within a week or two to prevent it from progressing. The way medicine is practiced these days, most people with a cancer diagnosis will have several weeks to gather information and make decisions about treatment, whether they want it or not, so take advantage of that time. If you don't have the research skills my friend has, find someone who does and ask for help. Some are listed in the Resources section.

You can find out about experimental trials for cancer at PDQ, a free service of the National Cancer Institute, at 800-422-6237. To assess other treatments, conventional or experimental for your type of cancer, do an Internet search or have someone who knows how do it for you. There are also numerous support groups, information groups about various kinds of cancer, and similar resources on the Web. You can search the National Library of Medicine database at www.pubmed.gov and download abstracts or articles on medical studies and research.

Besides making it more likely that you identify all your options, gathering information can prevent later regrets. When you know you've done good research you can make a decision without wishing you'd spent more time on it. For most people, information relieves anxiety and the feeling of being out of control—the more you know, the more active a role you can take in what happens to you.

Where else do you get good quality information? Unless you do not intend to explore what conventional Western medicine has to offer, start with your doctor. If you have a good relationship with a family doctor, an internist, or any M.D., ask if the doctor would be willing to work with you to gather and sort out information. Different opinions should ideally come from doctors from different medical groups, different cancer subspecialties (like radiation oncology, surgery, and medical oncology) and even different geographical areas, if possible. While this will take time and effort, it will let you know whether the recommended treatments are well accepted by the medical community. A wide variety of opinions indicates less certainty about the best way to proceed, thus your personal preferences and intuition may carry greater weight in your final decision.

As you talk with different experts you will be getting huge amounts of information about cancer and cancer treatment. Knowing that you have to absorb this complex new information under pressure can be overwhelming and confusing. It is unreasonable under the best of circumstances to think that you will become an expert in such a short time. But along with gathering information about treatment, you are gathering information about the doctors and cancer centers you visit. Pay attention to the values you hold important in treatment during these visits—how are you treated? How does the doctor and staff communicate? Who will be in charge of your treatment? How much access to that person will you have?

Most cancer patients today suffer not from a lack of information but an overdose of information. You can have trouble sorting it, evaluating it, and digesting it. Many of these decisions involve more than just knowing the statistics, and the help of a seasoned, knowledgeable, and caring cancer specialist can be invaluable to put everything into perspective.

When you consult with a doctor, write down your questions. They will change as you learn more about the illness and possible treatments. You won't remember everything so take a trusted friend or family member along to help you ask questions and remember what was said. Bring a tape recorder and ask the doctor if he or she minds if you tape the conversation for review later. Most doctors understand that a lot of information is covered and you won't be able to retain it all.

Several libraries specialize in information for cancer patients, like the Planetree Library in San Francisco. For a fee they will gather articles on your type of cancer and treatments from diverse sources, from medical journals to magazines and newspapers. Several commercial enterprises listed in the Resources section also provide information for a fee. I have often used the Moss Reports service to help my patients review possible complementary and alternative approaches to treatment. These services often give you access to ongoing research as time goes on.

Before long you'll probably accumulate a stack of books and articles so high you wouldn't be able to read them even if you wanted to. A few guides are particularly worthwhile. Perhaps the best is Michael Lerner's *Choices in Healing*, especially if you have a cancer that is not effectively treatable or where there is considerable difference of opinion in how to treat it. Lerner has made a long-term study of the issues people face as they attempt to choose the best cancer treatment, and he covers both conventional and alternative treatments. *The Complete Cancer Survival Guide* by Peter Teeley and Philip Bashe can give you fairly detailed information about how different types of common cancers are conventionally treated, and *Comprehensive Cancer Care: Integrating Alternative, Complementary and Conventional Therapies* by James Gordon, M.D., and Sharon Curtin offers a well-thought-out approach to these issues. Another book I highly recommend is *The Journey Through Cancer: An Oncologist's Seven-Level Program for Healing and Transforming the Whole Person* by Jeremy Geffen, M.D.

Books, however, especially those with detailed information on the medical treatment of cancer can be outdated by the time they are published due to the rapid emergence of new treatment approaches. That's one of the advantages to subscribing to a web-based service that is updated on a regular basis. With Web-interactivity, you can even request a search on a particular treatment approach or practitioner if the information is not listed.

Sorting Information

A challenge to modern cancer patients is that they often have too much information, and at the same time not enough. Too much in that they have stacks of books, tapes, newsletters, and articles, and too little in that they have no way to prioritize or sort the value of the information. Here are some tips to avoid getting overwhelmed:

1. Identify people who are good sources of information about cancer care in your community. These might be people with extensive experience in the field, a nurse, a doctor, a support group facilitator, or a cancer survivor who's been around the track a few times. Ask these people who they would see if they were in your position. If someone is recommended over and over again, or you are repeatedly told to avoid a certain party, that's valuable information.

Who you select as your main treatment person will be as important, and maybe more important than the kind of treatment you get, so gather as much background information as you can, and then set up consultations. A support group, whether local or a Web-based e-mail group, can serve as an excellent source of information for appropriate medical and self-care resources. Some are listed in the Resources section.

2. Ask for help from a friend or family member to help you sort and think through your options. Ask someone for help in organizing and filing your information if needed, and ask friends to be sounding boards to help you get clear on the best choices for you.

3. Go through the books, tapes, and papers you find fairly quickly, sorting them into three piles: (A) those you are definitely interested in and intend to read or research; (B) those you might be interested in at some later time; and (C) those that you wouldn't touch with a twenty-foot pole. Recycle or dispose of pile C, or donate it to your local cancer center or library. File the B pile. Then separate the A materials you have left into two piles: (1) possible treatment options and (2) self-healing materials.

4. Take these two piles and prioritize each one in order of what you think is most important.

5. Take the materials dealing with treatment options and, with the help of your support people, check the credentials of the source of information as best you can. Is this a credible person or organization? Does this person have a respected position in the cancer care community? Does the person publish and share findings? Is there a commercial interest or potential conflict of interest involved? Is the person accountable for his or her work? Is there a claim for a secret cure that you can only get from this person? If this pile is still too big, keep the most credible candidates and file the others away. Concentrate your research on the few you keep active.

6. Scan the self-care materials you have identified as the most important. Which ones are most accessible? Most easily read?

Listen to a tape from each series that attract you. Look for ones that help you relax, feel more positive, have suggestions that touch you, and leave you feeling better than you did before listening. Throw away any that irritate you, offend you, or are not compatible with your beliefs. Concentrate on those that help you develop the attitude you'd like to maintain during this time.

7. As you receive more materials, put them through the above process—are they of immediate interest? Of later interest? No interest whatsoever? Go through only those of immediate interest, evaluate their credibility, and decide if you want to pursue them further.

Get Multiple Opinions

Since cancer comprises many diseases, and since there is often more than one reasonable approach to treating many cancers, it is worth getting more than one opinion from cancer specialists in different medical groups. If you're fortunate and cost is no object, you may have a wide array of choices, and if not, you may be limited to a certain geographic area or even medical group. With guts and assertiveness, you may be able to get your local medical group to include treatment protocols that you find on your own, but this is hard work and demands persistence and an ability to negotiate and relate well with people under pressure. A friend or professional who acts as your *patient advocate* may be invaluable in such a situation. You might also decide that it's better for you to trust your doctors and let them do their work while you concentrate on your inner work and supportive nutritional and complementary therapies.

Complementary or Alternative Treatment

One decision you have the opportunity to make is whether or not to accept conventional medical treatment, add complementary therapies, or seek alternatives. As a physician who has long used complementary and alternative therapies in my practice, my advice is always to first determine what conventional treatment can offer you, then assess potential alternative treatments that seem viable. Use complementary treatments that make sense to you with whatever other treatment you choose.

Complementary treatments, as we have discussed, usually consist of improving your nutrition, reducing stress, doing exercises and movements, and employing adjuncts such as acupuncture, herbs, body and energy work aimed at increasing energy and vitality and supporting your immune system response. These complements are helpful in most circumstances. A well-nourished cancer patient will generally do better in all regards when compared to a malnourished cancer patient. A happy, relaxed, and focused patient will do better than an anxious, depressed, hopeless patient. Someone who feels relatively well during treatment is likely to do better, and certainly will feel better, than someone who is sick.

Many of my patients, using imagery, good nutrition, and traditional Chinese medicine are surprised that they feel as well as they do during their medical treatments. Of course, you need to assess carefully possible interactions between nutrients, herbs, and medications so that they don't cancel each other out, or worse. This is why having someone who is a knowledgeable source of both complementary and conventional treatment on your healing team is important.

Alternative treatment for cancer is another subject entirely. Rather than offering methods that augment or complement conventional treatments, these treatments claim to be effective as options in place of conventional treatments. This includes alternatives within the medical mainstream as well as alternatives outside of it. In my mind, truly alternative treatments are for consideration only if there is no good, reasonable, or acceptable conventional option, or if invasive and cytoreductive (cell-eliminating) therapies are just not acceptable.

The difficulty with the alternative cancer treatment arena is that it is even more difficult to tell what works and what doesn't than it is in conventional medicine. The types of research data available for conventional medicine aren't usually available for alternative medicine. The institutions of modern medicine deserve credit for making a concerted effort to discover whether what they do is of benefit or not, and they will change what they do according to the data in most cases. This capability has not been available to researchers in alternative medicine except in rare cases, although that is fortunately changing. Nevertheless, because this research is just beginning, you will rarely be able to look at good research data regarding alternative treatment approaches. Most data will be offered on the basis of a rationale, perhaps some animal research, and often just on the basis of testimonials.

People with cancer, especially those who have cancers with no good medical treatments, are notoriously vulnerable to fraudulent claims and expensive, worthless treatments. You will find hundreds to thousands of ways that people treat cancer, but usually without any substantial evidence that any of these alternative treatment choices are as effective as the usual course of treatment. They may pose less risk, although in many cases, safety studies haven't been done.

Traditional systems such as Chinese and Ayurvedic medicine can offer effective complementary treatments, but there is still little data from controlled studies to support their use as alternatives at this point.

My personal opinion is that if the evidence for conventional treatment is likely to provide you benefits that outweigh their risks, then use them, and further support your health with good nutrition, people and objects that are healing for you, and your inner game of healing. If conventional treatments do not meet this test, then seek alternatives that make sense, and support your own healing in the same ways.

How Physicians Evaluate Information about Cancer

It may be helpful to understand how physicians and scientists evaluate information about cancer treatments so you can evaluate their recommendations and create your own value-based hierarchy for sorting information.

The *Journal of the National Cancer Institute* employs a hierarchy system to sort through the immense amount of data and research they are asked to evaluate each year. Types of studies that produce the most reliable information are listed first, with less convincing forms of evidence following. Here is the order of hierarchy, in order of value:

Randomized double-blind placebo controlled studies: In this kind of research, groups of patients are assigned randomly to treatment or control groups, then matched by age, gender, and other criteria determined before the study. Treatments are administered by medical personnel who do not know whether the patient is getting the active treatment or "sham" placebo treatment. The treatment medications are manufactured to look exactly alike and coded so that the people giving the treatment are blind to what treatment they are giving. The patients also do not know whether they are getting placebo or experimental treatment (second level of blinding). At the end of the experiment, the data are analyzed to see if there is a difference between the treatment and control group. The codes are broken to see if one worked better than the other or had a different profile of adverse effects. If the treatment group has statistically better outcomes, and this outcome is repeated in other studies (replication), then this treatment usually enters into the realm of clinical choices for the oncologist and cancer patient.

The more often the replicated research shows the same outcome, the more reliable it is, so if a treatment consistently shows that 57 percent of the time patients go into remission, then those are the odds that it will work for you. Whether it actually will work for you or not is still unknown, since you are an individual, not a statistic. But what this kind of research shows is that the treatment itself has an effect on your type of cancer, above and beyond the effect of positive expectations (the placebo, or healing effect). The double-blind study design is extremely expensive and time-consuming, but is considered the gold standard for evaluating treatments.

Two things are especially important to understand about this type of research: first, you are not a statistic, and second, the power of the mind is so strong that we have to design experiments this complex and expensive in order to try to eliminate it from our assessments. As a person fighting for your health, you have a different goal than a researcher. While they want to eliminate the power of the mind, you want to *add* that power to your treatments.

Cohort studies: If double-blind controlled trials are not available, the next level of evidence are cohort trials, where a large number of people taking the treatment are observed. Since any treatment often has an expectation effect, cohort trials are interesting but inconclusive as to what part of the effect is from expectation and what part is from the treatment agent. However, if you have a cancer that is generally not highly treatable and a cohort trial is showing unusually good results, then it would be silly for you not to pay careful attention to that approach to treatment. A lot of the information available about traditional Chinese medicine over the past thirty years is from cohort trials.

Expert opinion: After cohort trials, we enter the realm of expert opinions, observation, and anecdotal case histories, which are often the only kind of evidence available about unproven and experimental treatments. In the medical world, treatments with such evidence behind them may be offered in clinical trials, whose designs have been approved by an Institutional Review Board to protect the rights of research subjects. There are different levels of such trials, from Phase 1 trials, whose goals are to see what toxicity the treatment has, through Phase 2 trials aimed at determining optimal dosages, to Phase 3 trials aimed at seeing how effective the treatment is in larger groups. Phase 4 trials further refine the dosage levels and allow for continued longer-term analysis of the treatment. Before conducting any of these human trials the treatment has usually gone through extensive testing on animals—and sometimes on humans in countries that are more liberal with their testing policies than the United States.

Rational mechanism: Sometimes there is no other evidence for a treatment than a compelling rationale or possible mechanism whereby a treatment could work. Unfortunately, there have been many good theoretical treatments for cancer that haven't worked for one reason or another, but it's better to have a rationale than take another step down and go to the pure "shots in the dark."

In an ideal world, we would have carefully controlled randomized double-blind trials for every option, accompanied by testing that could predict whether you as an individual are likely to benefit from a treatment. Unfortunately, we are far from this ideal in most circumstances, and you will be asked to make a decision based on incomplete and inconclusive data.

This is not easy. In the final analysis, you must make your decisions on whether you think a treatment is likely to do you more good than harm. The more harm the treatment can do, the more important it is that the treatment has good data to demonstrate that it can also do you good. A safe, nontoxic treatment is easy to choose if it makes sense to you and you can afford it. A risky, potentially toxic treatment demands more evidence of benefit.

In medicine, we call this the risk/benefit ratio. It's the best tool we have in a situation with so many variables. When assessing risk/benefit ratios you will notice that conventional cancer treatment usually carries a relatively high risk, when compared to natural approaches including nutrition, herbs, imagery, and so on, but in some cases it can yield a bigger benefit. If there is no good information on how likely it is a natural or alternative treatment will help, then part of the risk in choosing it as primary treatment includes the risk of *not* choosing a conventional treatment. For example, eating more vegetables is unlikely to cause you much harm, and may well do you some good, although there is slim if any evidence that it cures cancer all by itself. Chemotherapy might carry the risk of feeling ill, being temporarily vulnerable to infections, and suppressing immunity, but let's say it has a 60 percent cure rate for your type of cancer. If you chose vegetables over chemotherapy in this scenario, you'd have to consider the loss of a 60 percent chance of cure as part of the risk of that choice.

You'll generally find that complementary treatments, especially nutritional, mind-body-spirit, and exercise-related treatments carry little risk and potentially significant benefits, while medical and surgical treatments will carry larger risks. Because of the higher risks, the benefit should be substantially larger as well and these therapies more thoughtfully considered before adopting them.

With all these attempts to be as rational as possible, there are still many cancer treatment decisions that come down to factors that are personal, intuitive, and emotional:

Who do you trust?

Who and what are you most comfortable with?

Who and what do you think gives you the best shot to achieve your treatment goals?

How much discomfort and risk are you willing to tolerate?

Since these are not always easy questions, this is when guided imagery can help you clarify your thoughts and feelings. Once you have gathered your information and analyzed it to the best of your ability, there will come a time to choose, and your choice may not be obvious. If not, an imagery process can help you clarify your decision.

The script is called Crossroads Imagery with an Inner Healer. You'll imagine that in the company of a wise, kind guide who knows a lot about healing you walk different paths and imagine what the treatment results might be. Although you still need to be vigilant about how realistic certain fears may be, this imagery helps you look at options with both rationality and emotionality. This imagery brings intuitive as well as intellectual intelligence into the game. Ultimately, you want to make your choices from the wisest and most loving places you can, don't you?

Before you do Crossroads Imagery, make an effort to meet your Inner Healer or Advisor (see chapter 3). If for any reason this is not appropriate for you, then explore this imagery yourself—knowing that you can start and stop it anytime you want.

Crossroads Imagery with an Inner Healer

Take a comfortable position and let yourself begin to relax in your own way . . . let your breathing get a little deeper and fuller . . . but still comfortable . . . with every breath in, notice that you bring in fresh air, fresh oxygen, fresh energy that fuels your body . . . and with every breath out, imagine that you can release a bit of tension . . . a bit of discomfort . . . a bit of worry . . . and let that deeper breathing and the thoughts you have of fresh energy in and tension and worry out be an invitation to your body and mind to begin to relax . . . to begin to shift gears . . . and let it be an easy and natural movement . . . without having to force anything . . . without having to make anything happen right now . . . just letting it happen . . . just breathing and relaxing . . . breathing and energizing. . . .

Come back to taking a few deeper breaths whenever you feel like relaxing even more deeply . . . but for now, let your breathing take its own natural rate and its own natural rhythm . . . and simply let the gentle movement of your body as it breathes allow you to relax naturally and comfortably . . . almost without having to try. . . .

And noticing how your right foot feels right now . . . and how your left foot feels . . . and noticing that just before you probably weren't aware of your feet at all . . . but now that you turn your attention to them, you can notice them and how they feel . . . and notice the intelligence that is there in your feet . . . and notice what happens when you silently invite your feet to relax . . . and become soft and at ease . . . and in the same way noticing the intelligence in your legs and releasing your legs . . . and letting the intelligence in your legs respond in their own way . . . and noticing any release and relaxation that happens . . . without having to make any effort at all . . . just softening and releasing . . . and letting it be a comfortable and very pleasant experience. . . .

And you can relax even more deeply and comfortably if you want to . . . by continuing to notice the intelligence in different parts of your body and inviting them to soften and relax . . . and noticing how they relax . . . and you are in control of your relaxation and only relax as deeply as is comfortable for you . . . and if you ever need to return your awareness to the outer world you can do that by opening your eyes and looking around and coming fully alert . . . and if you need to respond to anything there you can do that . . . and knowing that you can do this if you need to . . . you can relax again and return your attention to the inner world of your imagination. . . .

Inviting the intelligence of your low back, pelvis, and hips to release and relax . . . and your abdomen and midsection . . . and your chest and rib cage . . . without effort or struggle . . . just letting go but staying aware as you do. . . inviting the intelligence in your back and spine to soften and release . . . in your low back . . . mid-back . . . between and across your shoulder blades . . . and across your neck and shoulders . . . the intelligence in your arms . . . and elbows . . . and forearms . . . through your wrists and hands . . . and the palms of the hands . . . the fingers . . . and thumbs. . . .

Noticing the intelligence in your face and jaws and inviting them to relax . . . to become soft and at ease . . . and your scalp and forehead . . . and your eyes . . . even your tongue can be at ease. . . .

And as you relax, let your attention shift from your usual outer world to what we can call your inner world . . . the world inside that only you can see, hear, smell, and feel . . . the world where your memories, your dreams, your feelings, your plans all reside . . . a world that you can learn to connect with . . . that can help you in many ways on your journey. . . .

And imagine that you find inside a very special place . . . a very beautiful place where you feel comfortable and relaxed, yet very aware . . . this may be a place that you have actually visited at some time in your life . . . in the outer world or even in this inner world . . . or it may be a place that you've seen somewhere . . . or it may be a brand-new place that you haven't visited before . . . and none of that matters as long as it is a very beautiful place, a place that invites you and feels good to be in . . . a place that feels safe and healing for you. . . .

And let yourself take some time to explore this place . . . and notice what you imagine seeing there . . . all the things you see . . . and how you see them . . . don't worry at all about how you imagine this place as long as it is beautiful to you and feels safe and healing . . . and notice if there are any sounds you imagine hearing . . . or if it is simply very quiet in your healing place . . . notice if there is a fragrance or aroma that you imagine there or a special quality of the air . . . there may or may not be, and it's perfectly all right however you imagine this place of healing . . . it may change over time as you explore it, or it may stay the same . . . it doesn't matter at this point . . . just let yourself explore a little more. . . .

Can you tell what time of day it is . . . or what time of year it is? . . . and what the temperature is like? . . . how you are dressed? . . . take some time to find a place where you feel safe

and let yourself get comfortable there . . . and just notice how it feels to imagine yourself there . . . and if your mind wanders from time to time, just take another deep breath or two and gently return your attention to this beautiful and healing place . . . just for now . . . without feeling the need to go anywhere else right now . . . or do anything else . . . just for now. . . .

And when you are ready, imagine starting out from your special safe place, walking on a road or path . . . walk for a while, noticing what you see, what you hear, what you smell, and how you feel as you walk along . . . let yourself feel connected to the earth beneath you and if you like, invite your Inner Healer or any guides, allies, or guardians you have to walk along with you . . . after some time, imagine that you come to a crossroads that has as many roads or paths branching off as you have treatments or treaters to choose from . . . pause for a little while and look as far down each road as you can see . . . notice what you see, or sense as you look down each road . . . pay attention to your feelings and body sensations as you do . . . notice whether you are attracted to one path more than the others, or if there is one or more that you feel repelled from or concerned about. . . .

When you are ready, discuss each path with your Inner Healer or Advisor, and see what it has to tell you about each path . . . and select one path to explore first. . . .

And let yourself move down this path in whatever way and whatever pace is suitable for you . . . trust your instincts as you explore, and notice what you observe as you move down the path . . . notice what you encounter, whether the path is easy or difficult . . . what kind of things you encounter on the path . . . if there are issues or obstacles to deal with . . . and notice how you might deal with them if you choose to . . . and how you proceed . . . and don't forget your Inner Healer if you need help or guidance . . . and see if there is an end to the path or not and if so, what is at the end of that path . . . or if it continues beyond where you can see or sense. . . .

When you are finished exploring that path, come back to the crossroads and take some time to review what you observed and noticed there . . . and then, depending on how you feel, you might either come back to your safe place, then to waking, and write or draw about what you observed on this path . . . or you might choose to explore another path in the same way . . . respect your-self and take whatever time you need . . . some people explore all the paths in one session . . . while others explore one path at a time and repeat the process some time later until they've explored each path in their imagery . . . either one is perfectly fine. . . .

And if you choose to explore another path now, go back one track on your CD and take the time to explore it . . . or if you are finished for now, prepare to bring back what you've learned into the outer world. . . .

And when you are ready, allow all the images to fade and go back within . . . knowing that healing continues to happen within you at all times . . . and gently bring your attention back to the room around you and the current time and place . . . and bring back with you anything that seems important or interesting to bring back, including any feelings of comfort, relaxation, or healing . . . and when you are all the way back, gently stretch and open your eyes. . . .

And take a few minutes to write or draw what you observed or sensed on each path . . . and take some time to compare your experience on each path . . . and perhaps to discuss it with anyone you feel close to.

Debriefing Your Experience

What did you notice on each path? Did different paths have different things waiting at the end, or were they similar? Which exploration was more comfortable? More interesting? More attractive?

Remember, this is a way to bring more of your intuition into a treatment decision when it isn't clear on a rational level what you should do. Notice what you learn from these explorations and what they mean to you in your decision-making process.

Answer these questions for each path you explored:

What did you experience on this path?

How did it feel traveling down this path?

What is your sense of what this path has to offer you?

What did your Inner Healer seem to think about this path? (Answer it if relevant.)

Once you've done this for each path, take some time answering the following questions:

What did you learn from exploring these paths ?

Are any of the paths compatible, or parallel, or do they lead to the same place?

Was this journey helpful in deciding which treatment course to pursue? If so, how?

You'll have lots of decisions to make as you go through your treatment, and you can always use this imagery process to help you decide what's likely to be best for you. The next three chapters will help you make the best use of medical, surgical, or radiation therapies if they are part of your treatment.

Summary

✦ Good medical decision making is a complex process involving gathering information, sorting information, obtaining multiple opinions, and using all your rational and intuitive abilities.

✦ Learning how doctors evaluate information can help you evaluate some of it for yourself.

✦ An imagery process can help you clarify your decision making, especially when the decisions are difficult.

7

Preparing for Successful Surgery

Numerous studies have shown that preparing for surgery with relaxation and imagery greatly reduces the time spent in the hospital, the degree of discomfort, and the frequency of postoperative complications. People preparing this way are less anxious, heal more quickly, and need fewer medications. I predict that guided imagery will soon be the standard of care in surgical preparation. A number of major insurance companies, including Blue Shield of California, PacifiCare of Arizona, and American Specialty Health Care, now routinely provide guided imagery tapes and self-care programs to patients before surgery because this practice clearly improves outcomes, saves money, and improves the experience for the patient. Blue Shield of California recently reported an average savings of $700 per surgical patient from using a guided imagery tape before surgery.[1] The financial savings may not be important to you, as the patient, but it translates into faster healing, less pain, and fewer complications, which does matter to you.

The remarkable research that has been conducted in this area is both exciting and encouraging. Henry Bennett and Elizabeth Disbrow are psychologists at the University of California at Davis who have found that if patients are simply told the day before surgery that they can have good outcomes, their outcomes improve. If specific suggestions to reduce common complications are made, patients tend to reduce significantly the frequency of such symptoms.

In one experiment, Disbrow and Bennett studied a group of patients about to have abdominal surgery. After this type of surgery, the bowels are sometimes affected, a complication called postoperative ileus that can be a serious, even life-threatening complication. The researchers visited these patients the day before surgery and told them that when they awoke in the recovery room, "your stomach will churn and growl, your intestines will pump and gurgle, and you will be hungry soon after surgery." They also asked patients about their favorite foods and suggested, "So that you can get back to eating your favorite food just as soon as possible, your stomach and intestines will start moving and churning and gurgling very soon after surgery." They found that patients instructed this way had 50 percent less ileus after their surgeries; their bowels moved in 2.6 days compared to an average of 4.2 days in the control group, who did not receive these instructions but were otherwise prepared identically.[2]

In an even more startling finding, Bennett and associates took another group of pre-surgical patients and discussed blushing as an example of how the body can shunt blood from one place to another. Then they gave them this suggestion: "Blood vessels are made of smooth muscle, and like any muscle, they contract or relax in localized areas to alter blood flow to the area. To make sure you will have very little blood loss in your surgery, it is very important that the blood move away from [the site of surgery] and out to other parts of the body during the operation. Therefore, the blood will move away from [the site of surgery] during the operation. Then, after your operation, it will return to that area to bring the nutrients to heal your body quickly and completely."

The patients they instructed in this way, just once, without any attempt to induce a hypnotic or trance state, lost an average 600cc of blood, compared to an average of 1100cc in the comparable control group who were not told that this was a possibility.[3] Other studies, using suggestions for improved immunity and quicker wound healing have also demonstrated positive effects to this simple, direct use of suggestion. Notice that all the suggestions are rich in imagery-laden language.

These and other studies routinely show that relaxation, encouragement, and instruction in recovery all have positive effects on surgical recovery. They also indirectly demonstrate what hypnotists have known for years—that people in stressful situations are highly suggestible, especially to suggestions from authority figures. Thus it is important for you to choose suggestions that are likely to be helpful, and be alert to those that aren't.

Unfortunately, many doctors are poorly trained in the effects of suggestion and unknowingly do harm with poor communication skills. A particularly relevant example is the customary preoperative "informed consent" procedure. Doctors have too often allowed this formality to become dictated by the concerns of attorneys. The result is often an unbalanced recitation of all the bad things that have ever happened to anyone, or that could possibly happen. The problem with this approach is that the statements about risks can act as unintended suggestions to the hypersuggestible if not counterbalanced by the positive aspects of the surgery, the reasons you decided on the procedure in the first place.

You of course need to know the risk associated with any procedure you choose, but when a rushed doctor delivers "informed consent" information the night or morning before surgery, dutifully reciting every bad thing that can possibly happen to a scared patient, I think it should be grounds for malpractice. The communication should instead take place long before the event and, most important, be counterbalanced with the potential benefits. If the benefits aren't likely to outweigh the risks, you shouldn't be having that procedure. The doctor should add, "You know, while these are real risks, most of the time these things do *not* happen, and the procedure goes well. This is why we've chosen to go ahead with this operation—do you still think this is the best choice for you? Good. Then let's both of us do everything we can to make sure that it is a success."

Once you've decided to have the operation, focus on having the best outcome. If your surgeon or anesthesiologist isn't aware of the power of positive imagery and suggestion, make sure that you take responsibility for it and aim to have the most successful treatment possible. Let your surgeon know that you have confidence in him or her and are working from the inside to help make the operation a success.

When preparing yourself for surgery it's important to know whether more or less information is helpful to you. Studies show two kinds of people in this regard: those who feel less anxious the more they know about something, and those who feel more anxious the more they know. People who need more information are sometimes called "vigilant copers" in the psychological literature—the more they know about what's going to happen with them, the better they feel. They do better knowing a good amount of detail about the surgery, the preoperative routine, and what to expect afterward. People who would rather not know so much are termed "avoidant copers"—they'd rather go to sleep and be awakened when it's over. If they are told too much about the process, they get more anxious. It's important to know that both methods work and there is no need to change your coping style in this situation. Honor your style and prepare accordingly.

If you are a vigilant coper, you'll want to make sure that all the questions you have about your surgery are answered either by the surgeon, the nurse, or staff. Ask for details you feel are important in your imagery of everything going well. You may have to be assertive to schedule time for this, but if you make it clear that you will be happy to pay for the time, you should be able to schedule it. Prepare for this meeting by writing down your questions to maximize your use of this time. If you have trouble getting in touch with your surgeon, fax your questions to the office and ask that someone knowledgeable get back to you in advance of your procedure.

If you do better with an avoidant style, concentrate on relaxation and waking up in recovery with everything having gone well. The script below allows you to use your own style. It includes details you think are important but also allows you to relax without adding detail, if that's more comfortable.

The first script, Preparing for a Successful Surgery, is for several days before your surgery. Listen to it as frequently as you like, and listen to it at least three to four times before the day of surgery. On the morning of surgery, listen to the second script, which is essentially the same, but rephrased in the appropriate tense for a surgery that day.

When you awaken in recovery, begin to listen to the third guided imagery script that follows, which will focus on comfort, rest, and the healing and recovery process. Listen to this exercise as frequently as you like, with a recommended frequency of one to three times daily while you are convalescing. In this script you are invited to form healing images that concentrate on recovery from surgery, but I have also included suggestions about healing the cancer, which can continue to support your focus on this most important process.

Preparing for Successful Surgery

Take a comfortable position and let yourself begin to relax in your own way . . . let your breathing get a little deeper and fuller . . . but still comfortable . . . with every breath in, notice that you bring in fresh air, fresh oxygen, fresh energy that fuels your body . . . and with every breath out, imagine that you can release a bit of tension . . . a bit of discomfort . . . a bit of worry . . . and let that deeper breathing and the thoughts you have of fresh energy in and tension and worry out be an invitation to your body and mind to begin to relax . . . to begin to shift gears . . . and let it be an easy and natural movement . . . without having to force anything . . . without having to make anything happen right now . . . just letting it happen . . . just breathing and relaxing . . . breathing and energizing. . . .

Come back to taking a few deeper breaths whenever you feel like relaxing even more deeply . . . but for now, let your breathing take its own natural rate and its own natural rhythm . . . and simply let the gentle movement of your body as it breathes allow you to relax naturally and comfortably . . . almost without having to try. . . .

And noticing how your right foot feels right now . . . and how your left foot feels . . . and noticing that just before you probably weren't aware of your feet at all . . . but now that you turn your attention to them, you can notice them and how they feel . . . and notice the intelligence that is there in your feet . . . and notice what happens when you silently invite your feet to relax . . . and become soft and at ease . . . and in the same way noticing the intelligence in your legs and releasing your legs . . . and letting the intelligence in your legs respond in their own way . . . and noticing any release and relaxation that happens . . . without having to make any effort at all . . . just softening and releasing . . . and letting it be a comfortable and very pleasant experience. . . .

And you can relax even more deeply and comfortably if you want to . . . by continuing to notice the intelligence in different parts of your body and inviting them to soften and relax . . . and noticing how they relax . . . and you are in control of your relaxation and only relax as deeply as is comfortable for you . . . and if you ever need to return your awareness to the outer world you can do that by opening your eyes and looking around and coming fully alert . . . and if you need to respond to anything there you can do that . . . and knowing that you can do this if you need to . . . you can relax again and return your attention to the inner world of your imagination. . . .

Inviting the intelligence of your low back, pelvis, and hips to release and relax . . . and your abdomen and midsection . . . and your chest and rib cage . . . without effort or struggle . . . just letting go but staying aware as you do. . . .

Inviting the intelligence in your back and spine to soften and release . . . in your low back . . . mid-back . . . between and across your shoulder blades . . . and across your neck and shoulders . . . the intelligence in your arms . . . and elbows . . . and forearms . . . through your wrists and hands . . . and the palms of the hands . . . the fingers . . . and thumbs. . . .

Noticing the intelligence in your face and jaws and inviting them to relax . . . to become soft and at ease . . . and your scalp and forehead . . . and your eyes . . . even your tongue can be at ease. . . .

And as you relax, let your attention shift from your usual outer world to what we can call your inner world . . . the world inside that only you can see, hear, smell, and feel . . . the world where your memories, your dreams, your feelings, your plans all reside . . . a world that you can learn to connect with . . . that can help you in many ways on your journey. . . .

And imagine that you find inside a very special place . . . a very beautiful place where you feel comfortable and relaxed, yet very aware . . . this may be a place that you have actually visited at some time in your life . . . in the outer world or even in this inner world . . . or it may be a place that you've seen somewhere . . . or it may be a brand-new place that you haven't visited before . . . and none of that matters as long as it is a very beautiful place, a place that invites you and feels good to be in . . . a place that feels safe and healing for you. . . .

And let yourself take some time to explore this place . . . and notice what you imagine seeing there . . . all the things you see . . . and how you see them . . . don't worry at all about how you imagine this place as long as it is beautiful to you and feels safe and healing . . . and notice if there are any sounds you imagine hearing . . . or if it is simply very quiet in your healing place . . . notice if there is a fragrance or aroma that you imagine there or a special quality of the air . . . there may or may not be, and it's perfectly all right however you imagine this place of healing . . . it may change over time as you explore it, or it may stay the same . . . it doesn't matter at this point . . . just let yourself explore a little more. . . .

Can you tell what time of day it is? . . . or what time of year it is? . . . and what the temperature is like? . . . how you are dressed? . . . take some time to find a place where you feel safe and let yourself get comfortable there . . . and just notice how it feels to imagine yourself there . . . and if your mind wanders from time to time, just take another deep breath or two and gently return your attention to this beautiful and healing place . . . just for now . . . without feeling the need to go anywhere else right now . . . or do anything else . . . just for now. . . .

And allow yourself to become aware of anything here that feels healing to you . . . it may be the beauty . . . it may be the sense of peacefulness . . . it may be the temperature, or the fragrance, or a combination of all the qualities that are here . . . perhaps you have a sense of what's sacred to you and what supports you in your life . . . it doesn't matter what you find healing here . . . or whether you can even identify it specifically . . . but let yourself experience whatever healing is there for you . . . and simply relax there . . . and know that while you relax, your body's natural healing systems can operate at their highest efficiency . . . without distraction . . . and without needing to be told what to do. . . .

The same built-in abilities to heal wounds, to repair injuries, to eradicate infections, and to destroy cancer cells that have been with you all your life can now function at full capacity . . . without any diversion of your precious energy . . . so while you relax, your body can take advantage of the time to fuel its ability to heal . . . as your muscles relax, your blood flows in all the right places . . . bringing your immune defenders to every place they are needed . . . and allowing them to efficiently and specifically target any cells that no longer belong to the healthy you . . . engulfing them and removing them . . . to be eliminated whenever you release what's no longer healthy for you . . . with your out breath . . . with your stool and urine . . . even with your sweat . . . and energizing yourself with fresh air and oxygen with every in breath . . . and with nutritious and healthy food . . . and with thoughts that bring you strength, courage, and even joy . . . and just letting yourself rest in this for a while. . . .

And from this place of deep relaxation and concentration, begin to focus on your intention to have an excellent outcome from your surgery . . . imagine the procedure going beautifully and that you recover rapidly and completely . . . remember that your doctors and nurses have spent most of their lives training and developing their skills so that they can be of service to you in this effort . . . imagine that on the day of surgery they are at their best, calm, focused, and at the top of their powers . . . you may also want to imagine in your own way that you are surrounded and protected by the love and good wishes of everyone whom you love and who loves you . . . and that any spiritual force or power you believe in is guiding and watching over you, now and during the procedure and recovery. . . .

And as you stay calm and relaxed throughout the surgery, your muscles can remain relaxed, making it easy for your doctor to do what needs to be done . . . you can be comfortable and at ease throughout . . . your blood pressure can remain steady as your muscles relax . . . while your muscles are relaxed it makes the whole procedure go more easily . . . the surgeon can see what needs to be seen . . . and anything that needs to be removed can come out easily . . . and afterward your muscles can heal quickly and completely. . . .

And while you are deeply relaxed, your body can move blood away from the site of surgery . . . all it needs to do is contract some of the blood vessels leading to the surgical site and open others to shunt it away . . . you don't even have to know how to do this, because your body already knows . . . just as it does when it blushes . . . and this makes it easy for the surgeon to see what needs to be seen . . . and easier to remove anything that needs to be removed. . . .

And when the procedure is over, your body can then return the blood flow to the affected areas and help them heal quickly and completely . . . bringing nutrients and oxygen . . . bringing special healing cells that make the repair . . . and immune defenders that scour the area clean and remove anything that doesn't belong there. . . .

When you wake up in the recovery room you may be surprised to notice that you'll be more comfortable and at ease than you would have imagined . . . but you can always ask for anything you need to become even more comfortable. . . .

When you wake up in the recovery room you may be surprised to find that it feels good to take a deep breath and clear your lungs . . . and as you come more clearly awake you may soon feel hungry . . . and start thinking about your favorite foods . . . your stomach and intestines may begin to gurgle and churn as you think about this. . . .

You may also be surprised to notice that you are more comfortable after surgery than you may have expected, and that you can handle any discomfort you feel . . . by relaxing deeply and allowing your body to heal. . . .

And because you're so relaxed, comfortable, and at ease, you find it easy to communicate with the staff and accept the good care they offer you . . . you can always ask your doctor, nurse, or a staff member for whatever you need to help you stay comfortable . . . and whenever you feel an urge to urinate you can find that easy to do. . . .

And you can continue to enjoy relaxing here for as long as you like . . . in this quiet, peaceful, beautiful place . . . with no need to go anywhere . . . and no need to do anything right now . . . except to relax . . . stay comfortable . . . and let your body heal as it knows so well how to do . . . if you'd like to take more time to focus on these positive thoughts and images, simply press the pause button on your audio player, and then press the play button when you are ready to go on. . . .

Taking all the time you need . . . and when you are ready to return your attention to the outer world, silently express any appreciation you might have for having a special healing place within you . . . and for being able to use your imagination in this way . . . and for the healing capabilities that have been built into you by nature . . . and when you are ready, allow all the images to fade and go back within . . . knowing that healing continues to happen within you at all times . . . and gently bring your attention back to the room around you and the current time and place . . . and bring back with you anything that seems important or interesting to bring back, including any feelings of comfort, relaxation, or healing . . . and when you are all the way back, gently stretch and open your eyes. . . .

And take a few minutes to write or draw about your experience.

Debriefing Your Experience

As usual, take some time to write or draw in your Healing Journal. If you haven't already, consider the following questions about your experience:

How do you feel after this process?
What was most interesting or important to you about this experience?

Is there anything else you'd like to include in your imagery about
your surgery? (If so, add it in each time you practice.)
Are there new questions for your surgical team that came to mind
while doing this imagery?

The next script is designed to be listened to on the day of surgery,
either before or after you take any preoperative medications. You can
play it as often as you like, and you can even ask a member of the medical staff to let you play it during surgery.

Some people believe that the unconscious responds to suggestions
even when you are anesthetized, though I feel the evidence is slim.
Nonetheless, it wouldn't hurt you if you choose to listen through surgery.

If you do play it during surgery, make sure your audio player has fresh
batteries, and adjust the volume to your comfort level before you receive
any preoperative medications. Protect your ears by taping the volume
control in position so it won't get changed during your procedure.

Successful Surgery Preparation: Day of Procedure

*Take a comfortable position and let yourself begin to relax in your own
way* ... let your breathing get a little deeper and fuller ... but
still comfortable ... with every breath in, notice that you literally
bring in fresh air, fresh oxygen, fresh energy that fuels your
body ... and with every breath out, imagine that you can release
a bit of tension ... a bit of discomfort ... a bit of worry ... and
let that deeper breathing and the thoughts you have of fresh
energy in and old energy out be an invitation to your body and
mind to begin to relax ... to begin to shift gears ... and let it be
an easy and natural movement ... without having to force anything ... without having to make anything happen right now ...
just breathing and relaxing ... breathing and energizing. ...

Come back to taking a few deeper breaths whenever you feel like relaxing even more deeply . . . but for now, let your breathing take its own natural rate and its own natural rhythm . . . and simply let the gentle movement of your body as it breathes allow you to relax naturally and comfortably . . . almost without having to try. . . .

And as you relax, let your attention shift from your usual outer world to what we can call your inner world . . . the world inside that only you can see, hear, smell, and feel . . . the world where your memories, your dreams, your feelings, your plans all reside . . . a world that you can learn to connect with . . . that can help you in many ways on your journey. . . .

And imagine once again that you find inside a very special place . . . a very beautiful place where you feel comfortable and relaxed, yet very aware . . . this may be a place that you have visited before . . . or it may be a place that you've seen somewhere . . . or it may be a brand-new place that you haven't visited before . . . and that doesn't matter as long as it is a very beautiful place, a place that invites you and feels good to be in . . . a place that feels safe and healing for you. . . .

And take some time to explore this place . . . and notice what you imagine seeing there today . . . all the things you see . . . and don't worry at all about how you imagine this place as long as it is beautiful to you and feels safe and healing . . . and notice if there are any sounds you imagine hearing . . . or if it is simply very quiet in your healing place . . . notice if there is a fragrance or aroma that you imagine there . . . there may or may not be, and it's perfectly all right however you imagine this place of healing . . . it may change over time as you explore it, or it may stay the same . . . it doesn't matter at this point . . . just let yourself explore a little more. . . .

Can you tell what time of day it is? . . . or what time of year it is? . . . and what the temperature is like? . . . and how you are dressed? . . . take some time to find a place where you feel safe and let yourself get comfortable there . . . and just notice how it feels to imagine yourself there . . . and if your mind wanders from time to time, just take another deep breath or two and gently return your attention to this beautiful and healing place . . . just for now . . . without feeling the need to go anywhere else right now . . . or do anything else . . . just for now. . . .

And allow yourself to become aware of anything here that feels healing to you . . . it may be the beauty . . . it may be the sense of peacefulness . . . it may be the temperature, or the fragrance, or a combination of all the qualities that are here . . . perhaps you have a sense of what's sacred to you and what supports you in your life . . . it doesn't matter what you find healing here . . . or whether you can even identify it specifically . . . but let yourself experience whatever healing is there for you . . . and simply relax there . . . and know that while you relax, your body's natural healing systems can operate at their highest efficiency . . . without distraction . . . and without needing to be told what to do. . . .

The same built-in abilities to heal wounds, to repair injuries, to eradicate infections, and to destroy cancer cells that have been with you all your life can now function at full capacity . . . without any diversion of your precious energy . . . so while you relax, your body can take advantage of the time to fuel its ability to heal . . . as your muscles relax, your blood flows in all the right places . . . bringing your immune defenders to every place they are needed . . . and allowing them to efficiently and specifically target any cells that no longer belong to the healthy you . . . engulfing them and removing them . . . to be eliminated whenever you release what's no longer healthy for you . . . with your out breath . . . with your stool and urine . . . even with your sweat . . . and energizing yourself with fresh air and oxygen with every in breath . . . and with nutritious and healthy food . . . and with thoughts that bring you strength, courage, and even joy . . . and just letting yourself rest in this for a while. . . .

And from this place of deep relaxation and concentration, begin to focus on your intention to have an excellent outcome from today's surgery . . . imagine the procedure going beautifully and that you recover rapidly and completely . . . remember that your doctors and nurses have spent most of their lives training and developing their skills so that they can be of service to you in this effort . . . imagine that on the day of surgery they are at their best, calm, focused, and at the top of their powers . . . you may also want to imagine in your own way that you are surrounded and protected by the love and good wishes of everyone who loves you . . . and that any spiritual force or power you believe in is guiding and watching over you, now and during the procedure and recovery. . . .

And as you stay calm and relaxed throughout the surgery, your muscles can remain relaxed, making it easy for your doctor to do what needs to be done . . . you can be comfortable and at ease throughout . . . your blood pressure can remain steady as your muscles relax . . . while your muscles are relaxed it makes the whole procedure go more easily . . . the surgeon can see what needs to be seen . . . and anything that needs to be removed can come out easily . . . and afterward your muscles can heal quickly and completely. . . .

And while you are deeply relaxed, your body can move blood away from the site of surgery . . . all it needs to do is contract some of the blood vessels leading to the surgical site and open others to shunt it away . . . you don't even have to know how to do this, because your body already knows . . . just as it does when it blushes . . . and this makes it easy for the surgeon to see what needs to be seen . . . and easier to remove anything that needs to be removed. . . .

And when the procedure is over, your body can then return the blood flow to the affected areas and help them heal quickly and completely . . . bringing nutrients and oxygen . . . bringing special healing cells that make the repair . . . and immune defenders that scour the area clean and remove anything that doesn't belong there. . . .

When you wake up in the recovery room you may be surprised to notice that you'll be more comfortable and at ease than you would have imagined . . . but you can always ask for anything you need to become even more comfortable. . . .

When you wake up in the recovery room you may be surprised to find that it feels good to take a deep breath and clear your lungs . . . and as you come more clearly awake you may soon feel hungry . . . and start thinking about your favorite foods . . . your stomach and intestines may begin to gurgle and churn as you think about this. . . .

You may also be surprised to notice that you are more comfortable after surgery than you may have expected, and that you can handle any discomfort you feel . . . by relaxing deeply and allowing your body to heal. . . .

And because you're so relaxed, comfortable, and at ease, you find it easy to communicate with the staff and accept the good care they offer you . . . you can always ask your doctor, nurse, or a staff member for whatever you need to help you stay comfortable . . . you may feel a gentle urge to urinate and find that easy to do. . . .

And you can continue to enjoy relaxing here for as long as you like . . . in this quiet, peaceful, beautiful place . . . with no need to go anywhere else . . . and no need to do anything right now . . . except to relax . . . stay comfortable . . . and let your body heal as it knows so well how to do. . . .

Taking all the time you need. . . .

Although this recording will stop in a few moments, it will begin again in a few minutes if you have set it to replay . . . or you can simply allow it to stop while you continue to stay relaxed and comfortable . . . remaining in this place for as long as you like, breathing easily, and enjoying how nice it feels to be in your special place, to relax, to dream, and to heal, until it's important for you to return your attention once more to the outer world . . . and when it is time to return your attention to the outer world, the staff will address you directly and when you hear them talking to you and asking you to come awake, you can begin to come awake, staying relaxed and comfortable as possible as you do . . . and already beginning to heal and recover . . . and feeling good about your ability to use your mind in this way to help you recover and heal.

This script is for you when you are recovering from your surgery. Play it soon after you awaken and as often as you like.

Guided Imagery for Healing after Surgery

Take a comfortable position and let yourself begin to relax in your own way . . . let your breathing get a little deeper and fuller . . . but still comfortable . . . with every breath in, notice that you bring in fresh air, fresh oxygen, fresh energy that fuels your body . . . and with every breath out, imagine that you can release a bit of tension . . . a bit of discomfort . . . a bit of worry . . . and let that deeper breathing and the thoughts you have of fresh energy in and tension and worry out be an invitation to your body and mind to begin to relax . . . to begin to shift gears . . . and let it be an easy and natural movement . . . without having to force anything . . . without having to make anything happen right now . . . just letting it happen . . . just breathing and relaxing . . . breathing and energizing. . . .

Come back to taking a few deeper breaths whenever you feel like relaxing even more deeply . . . but for now, let your breathing take its own natural rate and its own natural rhythm . . . and simply let the gentle movement of your body as it breathes allow you to relax naturally and comfortably . . . almost without having to try. . . .

And noticing how your right foot feels right now . . . and how your left foot feels . . . and noticing that just before you probably weren't aware of your feet at all . . . but now that you turn your attention to them, you can notice them and how they feel . . . and notice the intelligence that is there in your feet . . . and notice what happens when you silently invite your feet to relax . . . and become soft and at ease . . . and in the same way noticing the intelligence in your legs and releasing your legs . . . and letting the intelligence in your legs respond in their own way . . . and noticing any release and relaxation that happens . . . without having to make any effort at all . . . just softening and releasing . . . and letting it be a comfortable and very pleasant experience. . . .

And you can relax even more deeply and comfortably if you want to . . . by continuing to notice the intelligence in different parts of your body and inviting them to soften and relax . . . and noticing how they relax . . . and you are in control of your relaxation and only relax as deeply as is comfortable for you . . . and if you ever need to return your awareness to the outer world you can do that by opening your eyes and looking around and coming fully alert . . . and if you need to respond to anything there you can do that . . . and knowing that you can do this if you need to . . . you can relax again and return your attention to the inner world of your imagination. . . .

Inviting the intelligence of your low back, pelvis, and hips to release and relax . . . and your abdomen and midsection . . . and your chest and rib cage . . . without effort or struggle . . . just letting go but staying aware as you do. . . .

Inviting the intelligence in your back and spine to soften and release . . . in your low back . . . mid-back . . . between and across your shoulder blades . . . and across your neck and shoulders . . . the intelligence in your arms . . . and elbows . . . and forearms . . . through your wrists and hands . . . and the palms of the hands . . . the fingers . . . and thumbs. . . .

Noticing the intelligence in your face and jaws and inviting them to relax . . . to become soft and at ease . . . and your scalp and forehead . . . and your eyes . . . even your tongue can be at ease. . . .

And as you relax, let your attention shift from your usual outer world to what we can call your inner world . . . the world inside that only you can see, hear, smell, and feel . . . the world where your memories, your dreams, your feelings, your plans all reside . . . a world that you can learn to connect with . . . that can help you in many ways on your journey. . . .

And imagine that you find inside a very special place . . . a very beautiful place where you feel comfortable and relaxed, yet very aware . . . this may be a place that you have actually visited at some time in your life . . . in the outer world or even in this inner world . . . or it may be a place that you've seen somewhere . . . or it may be a brand-new place that you haven't visited before . . . and none of that matters as long as it is a very beautiful place, a place that invites you and feels good to be in . . . a place that feels safe and healing for you. . . .

And let yourself take some time to explore this place . . . and notice what you imagine seeing there . . . all the things you see . . . and how you see them . . . don't worry at all about how you imagine this place as long as it is beautiful to you and feels safe and healing . . . and notice if there are any sounds you imagine hearing . . . or if it is simply very quiet in your healing place . . . notice if there is a fragrance or aroma that you imagine there or a special quality of the air . . . there may or may not be, and it's perfectly all right however you imagine this place of healing . . . it may change over time as you explore it, or it may stay the same . . . it doesn't matter at this point . . . just let yourself explore a little more. . . .

Can you tell what time of day it is . . . or what time of year it is? . . . and what the temperature is like? . . . how you are dressed? . . . take some time to find a place where you feel safe and let yourself get comfortable there . . . and just notice how it feels to imagine yourself there . . . and if your mind wanders from time to time, just take another deep breath or two and gently return your attention to this beautiful and healing place . . . just for now . . . without feeling the need to go anywhere else right now . . . or do anything else . . . just for now. . . .

And allow yourself to become aware of anything here that feels healing to you . . . it may be the beauty . . . it may be the sense of peacefulness . . . it may be the temperature, or the fragrance, or a combination of all the qualities that are here . . . perhaps you have a sense of what's sacred to you and what supports you in your life . . . it doesn't matter what you find healing here . . . or whether you can even identify it specifically . . . but let yourself experience whatever healing is there for you . . . and simply relax there . . . and know that while you relax, your body's natural healing systems can operate at their highest efficiency . . . without distraction . . . and without needing to be told what to do. . . .

The same built-in abilities to heal wounds, to repair injuries, to eradicate infections, and to destroy cancer cells that have been with you all your life can now function at full capacity . . . without any diversion of your precious energy . . . so while you relax, your body can take advantage of the time to fuel its ability to heal . . . as your muscles relax, your blood flows in all the right places . . . bringing your immune defenders to every place they are needed . . . and allowing them to efficiently and specifically target any cells that no longer belong to the healthy you . . . engulfing them and removing them . . . to be eliminated whenever you release what's no longer healthy for you . . . with your out breath . . . with your stool and urine . . . even with your sweat . . . and energizing yourself with fresh air and oxygen with every in breath . . . and with nutritious and healthy food . . . and with thoughts that bring you strength, courage, and even joy . . . and just letting yourself rest in this for a while. . . .

Now that your surgery is completed, you can focus on thoughts and images that can help make your recovery more comfortable . . . and continue to encourage the healing ability of your body and mind . . . your body is always actively involved in the healing and recovery process and this is a time when you can support that healing by relaxing, getting the rest you need, eating well, and using the same ability to relax and imagine that has helped you before. . . .

Remember that your body knows how to heal, as it has many times before . . . and you may want to recall all the times you may have suffered a cut or bruise . . . or burn . . . or a cold or other illness or injury that you eventually recovered from . . . and how amazing it is that your body knew just what to do to repair the injury or wound . . . or to eradicate the infection . . . or to heal from the illness . . . so it knows what to do . . . and it has already begun that natural process of healing . . . your blood is constantly circulating, bringing fresh oxygen and nutrients, immune cells, and other special repair cells that know exactly where to go and what to do in order to help you heal completely and well. . . .

While you heal, you may require more rest than you normally do as your body directs energy and resources to the area that is actively healing . . . by giving yourself that rest, you are helping yourself to a faster and more complete recovery . . . and as your body heals, you can feel more and more comfortable . . . and you can enhance your comfort levels and speed your recovery by listening to this tape. . . .

You can listen as often as you like, any time during the day or night . . . the more you relax and imagine the healing you desire, the more energy your body can put into healing . . . listen to it at least once a day until you are completely recovered. . . .

And take a moment to focus on the areas of your body that are actively healing, repairing, and strengthening themselves now . . . imagine the blood flowing easily and freely through all those areas . . . the fresh red blood bringing all the oxygen, energy, repair cells, nutrients, and other materials that the body uses for rapid and healthy repair. . . .

As the blood delivers nutrients and healing elements, it also washes away any waste products, any inflammation, any swelling or discomfort, and anything else that doesn't belong there . . . leaving the area behind cleansed, renewed, vibrant, and healing beautifully. . . .

As the body brings itself back into wholeness it brings special attention to any area needing repair . . . healing itself in such a way that it becomes even stronger in that area than it was before. . . .

And as your body heals, imagine yourself having a full and complete recovery . . . working with your body and mind to build strength and resiliency. . . .

Imagine the ways that you can help create a level of health and well-being that may be even better than the one you had before surgery . . . and how you can make the best use of the process of healing you are now going through . . . looking forward to moving and using your body actively again.

Notice any feelings of pleasure you get as you imagine yourself feeling better and better, and allow those feelings to grow stronger as they expand throughout your body and mind. . . .

Imagine the things you may be able to do when you are better . . . especially the things you most love to do . . . and imagine doing them with whomever you love to do them with . . . there may even be things you haven't been able to do for a while . . . and some may be things you'll be able to do when you recover . . . if there are things you can no longer do, imagine some other things you'd like to do that you didn't have time for before. . . .

And if there are any good feelings that come with imagining yourself this way, let yourself feel them as fully as you can . . . and enjoy them as fully as you can. . . .

If you want to continue to imagine the best results of the healing process for a while longer, simply ignore the invitation I am about to give you to return to waking . . . or press the pause button on your player. . . .

And release it or press the play button when you are ready to come back to awareness of the outer world . . . or if you prefer, just let yourself doze off and sleep . . . letting the deep restfulness further support your healing. . . .

(Pause for 10 seconds)

Now prepare yourself to come back to your outer world . . . and when you come awake, you can feel awake and alert, and good about yourself and the ways you are using the power of your mind to support your healing. . . .

And begin now to notice what is going on in the outer world around you and gently bring your full attention back to the outer world . . . become aware of what you hear around you . . . and as you open your eyes, of what you see . . . and as you come back to the outer world you can feel refreshed . . . and comfortable . . . and bring back anything that seems important to bring back . . . taking all the time you need to come fully aware . . . feeling better than before . . . and knowing you can go back into this deep comfortable state anytime you feel like it. . . .

When you are fully awake, and if you feel like it, you may want to write or draw about this experience in your Healing Journal.

Debriefing Your Experience

Once you've written or drawn about your experience in your Healing Journal, answer the following questions, if you haven't already.

What do you notice about the way you imagine the process of healing?
How does your healing seem to be progressing?
Is there anything that seems to be missing that would help you heal even faster and more completely?
What might it be like to provide that, or imagine providing that?
Do you have any other thoughts or questions about your healing that you'd like answered?

Summary

+ Mentally preparing for surgery has been shown to reduce pain, complications, bleeding, and time spent in the hospital.

- Knowing how to mentally prepare yourself for surgery can help protect you from inadvertent suggestions about risks.
- Guided imagery is a well-proven method for mentally preparing for a successful surgery.
- Listening to tapes before and after surgery is extremely useful. You can even have them playing during surgery with permission of your surgeon and anesthesiologist.

8

Making the Most of Chemotherapy

Chemotherapy is the use of strong medicines to destroy cancer cells. About a third of chemotherapy agents are derived from natural sources; others have been created in the laboratory. While different chemotherapy drugs have different mechanisms, most of them are cellular poisons that typically interfere with a cell's ability to divide and grow. Since cancer cells divide faster than normal cells they have a faster metabolic rate and take in an inordinate share of what comes to them in the bloodstream. This includes chemotherapy agents, so abnormal cells suffer much more than normal cells when these drugs are taken. In certain cancers, chemotherapy is curative, while in others it weakens the cancer and gives the natural defenses a chance to overcome it. In still other forms of cancer, chemotherapy is called an *adjuvant* treatment, meaning it is given as an additional precaution against the return of cancer by eliminating possible microscopic areas of cancer after surgery or radiation.

If chemotherapy is appropriate for the type of cancer you have, then it can help you in your fight. Chemotherapy is not without risk, with potential toxicity to the heart, nervous system, and immune system being the most significant. Because immune cells are also rapidly dividing cells, they frequently suffer from the effects of chemotherapy. That's why it's important to carefully weigh the potential benefits against the risks before choosing chemotherapy. In effect, you're bombing your own troops as well as the enemy and you need to make sure it's worth it.

Because American culture is so deeply ingrained with the idea that medicine is synonymous with drugs, and because we are so afraid of cancer, chemotherapy sometimes is recommended in situations where it is of questionable value. Because we have so little real scientific data on medical approaches to cancer treatment other than chemotherapy, it may be offered as "the best we have" by conventional physicians. Many doctors and people are afraid of "doing nothing" when cancer is involved, and because natural or alternative treatments for cancer are unproven, they are often wrongly considered to be "nothing." Declining chemotherapy when the risks outweigh the benefits is a rational treatment choice that is too often ignored.

In many cases, however, chemotherapy is a useful part of cancer treatment. If you decide to have chemotherapy it is clearly in your interest to make the best of it. I encourage you to imagine it doing exactly what you'd want it to do, with minimal or no side effects. This has been shown to reduce adverse effects, and I believe that in the future we will be able to demonstrate that it makes the treatment more effective as well.

The great bulk of research on the placebo effect demonstrates that expectations have significant effects on treatments, whether they are surgical, medical, or psychological. Remarkable animal research shows that when an animal expects to have a certain immune response to a substance, it activates the response itself. This research, by Dr. Robert Ader and his colleagues at Rochester University, catapulted the new science of psychoneuroimmunology (PNI) into medical respectability about fifteen years ago, when these findings were first reported. Ader took mice and gave them saccharine-sweetened water containing an immune-suppressing medicine (cyclophosphamide). After a while the researchers counted the circulating immune cells of the mice and predictably found that the mouse immune system had been suppressed to a certain extent. After a number of exposures to the flavored water containing the drug, they simply gave the mice the saccharine-flavored water and found that, even without any medication included, the mice suppressed their own immune systems about 50 percent as much as when they were given the drug.[1]

The immune system seems to be a fast learner. Which is all the more reason that we should begin doing immune-stimulating imagery as soon as we find out we are fighting cancer. If we have even a week or two head start, we have a chance of stimulating the system through imagery to maintain immune function while taking chemotherapy. And when you consider that imagery has been shown to relieve anxiety, depression, and nausea associated with chemotherapy, it makes it an invaluable tool.

Fully one-quarter to one-third of people get nauseous and vomit just thinking about chemotherapy, so the role of the mind in side effects is important and real. This is, of course, an unguided—or perhaps misguided—use of imagery and, predictably, anticipatory nausea and vomiting responds well to relaxation and positive imagery.[2]

Other studies examining the effects of guided imagery and hypnosis, which essentially consists of relaxation and imagery-laden suggestions, have also demonstrated success in reducing or eliminating anticipatory and/or post-treatment nausea in both adults and children.[3] Fortunately, advances have also been made in medical treatment of nausea and vomiting that may accompany chemotherapy, and the combination of the new medications and guided imagery is even better than either used alone.

In a study conducted at the Arthur G. James Cancer Hospital and Research Institute, patients using chemotherapy-specific guided imagery reported a "significantly more positive experience."[4] Another study in the *British Journal of Cancer* reported on 96 breast cancer patients who used guided imagery and relaxation for their chemotherapy. Patients were more relaxed during chemotherapy, and had a better quality of life, leading the study's authors to conclude that relaxation and guided imagery were "simple, inexpensive and beneficial" for patients undergoing chemotherapy.[5]

This quality of experience has significant clinical effects, because as many as 31 percent of chemotherapy patients prematurely terminate treatment due to anxiety or depression alone.[6] If you are able to finish your prescribed course of treatment, the odds of it being successful go way up.

Imagery can also help with other chemotherapy related problems. A 1995 study published in the journal *Pain* demonstrated that imagery, relaxation, and cognitive behavioral training can reduce the pain of mouth sores, a common side effect from some types of chemotherapy.[7]

The guided imagery script below was tested at the UCSF–Mount Zion Cancer Center in San Francisco. A pilot study showed that anxiety associated with chemotherapy was relieved at the first listening. In it you will have the opportunity to imagine elements of healing that are helpful to people going through or anticipating chemotherapy. Although it's a structured process, you will have the opportunity to imagine each of these elements in your own way. Don't worry about whether the way you imagine them is "right" or not—it's a waste of time. It has not been shown that one image is better than another—your own imagery is the most powerful. Imagine each process in your own way and affirm that your unconscious healing abilities understand what you are encouraging them to do.

Since we don't yet know what type of imagery is best for each individual, the script presents four important elements of healing:

1. Deep relaxation, in which the natural healing elements of your body work at their best, protecting the normal and healthy cells, especially those that are most vulnerable and that you are concerned about.
2. Imagining the chemotherapy medications effectively and completely destroying any cancer cells.

3. Imagining an aggressive immune response mopping up any debris or remaining cancer cells in whatever condition they are found.
4. Imagining yourself enjoying the benefits of a successful treatment, doing the things you love to do with the people you love to do them with.

Listen to this guided imagery script a few times and see what imagery comes up for you. Your imagery may change or evolve as you practice with the script. This is normal. Notice how your imagery changes, if it does, as you imagine your chemotherapy doing its work. Imagine your healing happening as if you could really make it happen that way. No wishing, hoping, or begging, just imagine that it works exactly the way you'd like it to work. Concentrate on the elements that are most helpful, meaningful, or powerful to you.

You can use this imagery process to prepare yourself before chemotherapy by using it once or twice a day for a week beforehand. Then do it frequently during the time you are receiving the chemotherapy and for the five days following each treatment.

Making the Most of Chemotherapy

Take a comfortable position and let yourself begin to relax in your own way . . . let your breathing get a little deeper and fuller . . . but still comfortable . . . with every breath in, notice that you bring in fresh air, fresh oxygen, fresh energy that fuels your body . . . and with every breath out, imagine that you can release a bit of tension . . . a bit of discomfort . . . a bit of worry . . . and let that deeper breathing and the thoughts you have of fresh energy in and tension and worry out be an invitation to your body and mind to begin to relax . . . to begin to shift gears . . . and let it be

an easy and natural movement . . . without having to force anything . . . without having to make anything happen right now . . . just letting it happen . . . just breathing and relaxing . . . breathing and energizing. . . .

Come back to taking a few deeper breaths whenever you feel like relaxing even more deeply . . . but for now, let your breathing take its own natural rate and its own natural rhythm . . . and simply let the gentle movement of your body as it breathes allow you to relax naturally and comfortably . . . almost without having to try. . . .

And noticing how your right foot feels right now . . . and how your left foot feels . . . and noticing that just before you probably weren't aware of your feet at all . . . but now that you turn your attention to them, you can notice them and how they feel . . . and notice the intelligence that is there in your feet . . . and notice what happens when you silently invite your feet to relax . . . and become soft and at ease . . . and in the same way noticing the intelligence in your legs and releasing your legs . . . and letting the intelligence in your legs respond in their own way . . . and noticing any release and relaxation that happens . . . without having to make any effort at all . . . just softening and releasing . . . and letting it be a comfortable and very pleasant experience. . . .

And you can relax even more deeply and comfortably if you want to . . . by continuing to notice the intelligence in different parts of your body and inviting them to soften and relax . . . and noticing how they relax . . . and you are in control of your relaxation and only relax as deeply as is comfortable for you . . . and if you ever need to return your awareness to the outer world you can do that by opening your eyes and looking around and coming fully alert . . . and if you need to respond to anything there you can do that . . . and knowing that you can do this if you need to . . . you can relax again and return your attention to the inner world of your imagination. . . .

Inviting the intelligence of your low back, pelvis, and hips to release and relax . . . and your abdomen and midsection . . . and your chest and rib cage . . . without effort or struggle . . . just letting go but staying aware as you do. . . .

Inviting the intelligence in your back and spine to soften and release . . . in your low back . . . mid-back . . . between and across your shoulder blades . . . and across your neck and shoulders . . . the intelligence in your arms . . . and elbows . . . and forearms . . . through your wrists and hands . . . and the palms of the hands . . . the fingers . . . and thumbs. . . .

Noticing the intelligence in your face and jaws and inviting them to relax . . . to become soft and at ease . . . and your scalp and forehead . . . and your eyes . . . even your tongue can be at ease. . . .

And as you relax, let your attention shift from your usual outer world to what we can call your inner world . . . the world inside that only you can see, hear, smell, and feel . . . the world where your memories, your dreams, your feelings, your plans all reside . . . a world that you can learn to connect with . . . that can help you in many ways on your journey. . . .

And imagine that you find inside a very special place . . . a very beautiful place where you feel comfortable and relaxed, yet very aware . . . this may be a place that you have actually visited at some time in your life . . . in the outer world or even in this inner world . . . or it may be a place that you've seen somewhere . . . or it may be a brand-new place that you haven't visited before . . . and none of that matters as long as it is a very beautiful place, a place that invites you and feels good to be in . . . a place that feels safe and healing for you. . . .

And let yourself take some time to explore this place . . . and notice what you imagine seeing there . . . all the things you see . . . and how you see them . . . don't worry at all about how you imagine this place as long as it is beautiful to you and feels safe and healing . . . and notice if there are any sounds you imagine hearing . . . or if it is simply very quiet in your healing place . . . notice if there is a fragrance or aroma that you imagine there or a special quality of the air . . . there may or may not be, and it's perfectly all right however you imagine this place of healing . . . it may change over time as you explore it, or it may stay the same . . . it doesn't matter at this point . . . just let yourself explore a little more. . . .

Can you tell what time of day it is? . . . or what time of year it is? . . . and what the temperature is like? . . . how you are dressed? . . . take some time to find a place where you feel safe and let yourself get comfortable there . . . and just notice how it feels to imagine yourself there . . . and if your mind wanders from time to time, just take another deep breath or two and gently return your attention to this beautiful and healing place . . . just for now . . . without feeling the need to go anywhere else right now . . . or do anything else . . . just for now. . . .

And allow yourself to become aware of anything here that feels healing to you . . . it may be the beauty . . . it may be the sense of peacefulness . . . it may be the temperature, or the fragrance, or a combination of all the qualities that are here . . . perhaps you have a sense of what's sacred to you and what supports you in your life . . . it doesn't matter what you find healing here . . . or whether you can even identify it specifically . . . but let yourself experience whatever healing is there for you . . . and simply relax there . . . and know that while you relax, your body's natural healing systems can operate at their highest efficiency . . . without distraction . . . and without needing to be told what to do. . . .

The same built-in abilities to heal wounds, to repair injuries, to eradicate infections, and to destroy cancer cells that have been with you all your life can now function at full capacity . . . without any diversion of your precious energy . . . so while you relax, your body can take advantage of the time to fuel its ability to heal . . .

as your muscles relax, your blood flows in all the right places . . . bringing your immune defenders to every place they are needed . . . and allowing them to efficiently and specifically target any cells that no longer belong to the healthy you . . . engulfing them and removing them . . . to be eliminated whenever you release what's no longer healthy for you . . . with your out breath . . . with your stool and urine . . . even with your sweat . . . and energizing yourself with fresh air and oxygen with every in breath . . . and with nutritious and healthy food . . . and with thoughts that bring you strength, courage, and even joy . . . and just letting yourself rest in this for a while. . . .

As you are enjoying this comfortable state, begin to imagine that any treatment you are going to receive will work perfectly for you . . . research has already shown that imagining your treatment working well can add to its positive benefits. . . .

Before your treatment begins, you can direct your intention by imagining that you are protecting the healthy cells of your body, especially your hair, your digestive tract, your bone marrow, your heart, and any other areas of your body that don't need to receive the effects of the medication . . . you might imagine that you turn down the supply of blood to your healthy tissues while you are receiving the chemotherapy . . . just imagine that before the chemotherapy the blood supply is temporarily shut down to healthy areas of your body, leaving just enough to maintain them in good health . . . you might imagine closing valves at appropriate places, or just having a computer-controlled system that not only shuts down the blood supply to healthy tissues, but at the same time directs the great bulk of your bloodstream along with the chemotherapy medication directly to the areas of your body that really need it, any tissues or cells that are abnormal and need to be destroyed . . . you can imagine that the healthy tissues are protected by a shield or a powerful white light . . . a spiritual or protective force . . . or an energy screen that shelters them from the medication . . . as if you can wall off and protect any healthy tissues in your body while the chemotherapy floods any cancer cells or tissues . . . let yourself imagine this protection in whatever way it comes to you . . . pay special attention to your scalp and imagine that you shunt most of the blood away from your stomach and intestines temporarily . . . and set up a filter or a shield inside and around your heart so that medications are pumped through it to the areas in your body that really need it, without being absorbed by your heart . . . that the cells in the marrow of your bones where your new blood cells are made are protected and shielded from the medication . . . and imagine that you can guide the medication directly to the areas of your body that need the medication. . . .

Imagine that as the medication reaches cancer cells it kills them rapidly, effectively, and completely . . . you might imagine them exploding, imploding, melting, shriveling, drying up, or in some other way . . . maybe you have your own image and that's even better . . . just imagine the chemotherapy doing exactly what it's meant to do, and destroying cancer cells . . . whether you imagine a dramatic death as above or the medication turns them into good little spirits and sends them to heaven doesn't matter . . . imagine it happening anyway you imagine it . . . but do it right . . . completely . . . imagine it working exactly as you'd like it to—concentrating on eradicating cancer . . . and leaving the healthy cells alone . . . and if there's anything you have gained by having cancer, anything you've learned that you appreciate, affirm that you can keep what's healthy while letting go of what's not. . . .

Now that any abnormal cells are weakened or destroyed, imagine a vigorous and ebullient response from your immune defense system . . . imagine billions and billions of immune cells, killer cells, swarming into the area being treated and wiping up any remaining cancer cells, debris, and chemical residue of the battle and reestablishing a healthy, controlled, well-organized environment into which healthy cells can once again grow . . . they are cleaning up the neighborhood and making it safe once again for good health . . . imagine that there are many hundreds of thousands as many immune cells as cancer cells (because there are), and that they can now easily identify and overcome any remaining cells . . . imagine the cancer cells dead, badly injured, and dazed . . . disorganized and completely vulnerable to the aggressive and highly motivated immune cells . . . give your immune cells a cheer and let them know how much you are behind them . . . root them on! . . . maybe there's a cavalry charge sounding in the background . . . maybe there's some other music or some battle cry that they have . . . pour it on . . . imagine that they are efficient, aggressive, and without hesitation remove any cells that are not functioning in healthy cooperation with their neighbors and their function in the whole person . . . a lot of energy goes into this . . . and imagine that your immune system will remain strong and powerful throughout . . . on the job twenty-four hours a day . . . waking or sleeping . . . and that every time you check in on them and support them this way it encourages them to fight on. . . .

Take some time to notice what it feels like to have these powerful combined forces on your side. . . .

Now imagine that you move into the future . . . sometime in the not too distant future when your chemotherapy treatment is all over and you have had the very best outcome you can imagine . . . and that you are once again doing the things that you enjoy . . . with the people you enjoy doing them with . . . and enjoying a restored sense of good health. . . .

Imagine that you are feeling very good about making the best use of your treatment and getting the very best results from it . . . having the treatment work just the way that you imagine it working . . . and feeling very good about it.

And imagine yourself in the future, on a date you want to see, visiting your doctor and your doctor smiling, giving you good news . . . see the date on the wall . . . both you and your doctor feeling very, very good about the successful treatment you have received . . . and seeing yourself as far into the future as you'd like to imagine yourself, doing things that are meaningful and enjoyable to you . . . and feeling very grateful that you are able to get good treatment and make the very best use of it. . . .

Taking all the time you need. . . .

And when you are ready to return your attention to the outer world, silently express any appreciation you might have for having a special healing place within you . . . and for being able to use your imagination in this way . . . and for the healing capabilities that have been built into you by nature . . . and when you are ready, allow all the images to fade and go back within . . . knowing that healing continues to happen within you at all times . . . and gently bring your attention back to the room around you and the current time and place . . . and bring back with you anything that seems important or interesting to bring back, including any feelings of comfort, relaxation, or healing . . . and when you are all the way back, gently stretch and open your eyes. . . .

And take a few minutes to write or draw about your experience.

Debriefing Your Experience

As usual, write or draw what seemed significant or interesting to you about this experience. Following that, answer the following, if you haven't already:

How do you feel after doing this process?

How did you imagine protecting your healthy cells? How might you in the future?

How did you imagine the chemotherapy medication? How did you imagine directing it to the cancer cells, and how did they react when the chemotherapy came in contact?

How might this be imagined even more powerfully in the future?

How did you imagine your immune response?

How might this be imagined even more powerfully in the future?

How did you imagine yourself in the future?

How did you look?

How far in the future was this?

What were you doing?

Who were you with?

Are there other future images that would also bring positive motivation to you?

What seemed most important or interesting to you about your imagery this time?

Summary

* When chemotherapy is well chosen, it is powerful medicine. Its benefits need to be measured against its risks.
* Many people discontinue chemotherapy prematurely because of anticipating side effects. Imagery can help prevent this.
* Guided imagery can reduce or eliminate emotional and physical side effects of many chemotherapy regimens and allow you to make the best use of them.

❖

9

Making the Most of Radiation Therapy
and Other Treatments

Radiation therapy is the third cancer-killing treatment commonly used in medicine. In some cases, it can be curative, and in others it can buy you time, relieve pain, and protect vulnerable and critical organs from cancer damage. Like surgery and chemotherapy, it is not without risks, depending on how much radiation you receive, how well focused it is, and what organs will be affected by it. Most people undergoing a significant course of radiation therapy are fatigued for a while after the treatment, and some will experience side effects from tissues that are affected—nausea or diarrhea if the bowel is irradiated, trouble with salivation if the salivary glands are affected, and so on.

There is less research evidence that guided imagery is helpful for radiation than for surgery or chemotherapy, but the evidence that exists is consistent and positive. A recent study in the journal *Oncology Nursing Forum* reported that women receiving radiation treatment for Stage 1 and 2 breast cancer were significantly more comfortable during therapy when they listened to a guided imagery audiotape once daily.[1] A literature review published in the *Journal of the National Cancer Insti-*

tute, reported that "fifty-four published studies using a variety of research designs were identified for review.... Behavioral intervention integrating several behavioral methods can ameliorate anxiety and distress associated with invasive medical treatments.[2] This is consistent with all the data we have about using guided imagery before, during, and after any medical intervention, including MRI, colonoscopy, angiography, surgery, and chemotherapy.

Christopher Sato-Perry, a Ph.D. candidate in psychology, has conducted 3,000 Interactive Guided Imagery[sm] sessions with more than 250 patients undergoing radiation for cancer treatment. Working at the Radiation Oncology Center of California Pacific Medical Center (CPMC) in San Francisco, Sato-Perry teaches his patients to relax and to find a way to positively imagine the treatment. Interestingly, this may involve a dialogue or negotiation with an image of the treatment or an image of the nausea or fatigue. Sato-Perry believes, as I do, that this is often the most powerful way to use imagery, because it evokes highly personal imagery—which tends to have the most powerful effect on any individual.

At CPMC, sessions are offered to everyone who undergoes radiation therapy. Brochures in the waiting room describe the guided imagery program as an integral part of the treatment. Sato-Perry reports that approximately 20 percent of the patients take advantage of the guided imagery program, and 19 out of 20 patients who have one session go on to finish six sessions. Doctors, nurses, and staff see how useful it is to people, and most have experienced guided imagery themselves, courtesy of Sato-Perry. Dr. Mark Rounsaville, a CPMC radiation oncologist, has been a vocal supporter of the program, saying, "It's clear that patients need a lot more than radiation, surgery, and chemotherapy treatment. Their psychological and spiritual needs must also be recognized and tended to. Cancer can be the challenge of a lifetime and patients need to be shown how to harness all their capabilities to get through the diagnosis, treatment, and recovery. Interactive Guided Imagery[sm] sessions should be prescribed while treating cancer in the same manner as one prescribes medication."

Mike, a burly man in his late fifties, was diagnosed with Stage 4 lung cancer. A labor negotiator from Chicago and a lifetime smoker and drinker, Mike was the salt of the earth and not the type of person you'd think would embrace guided imagery. He received radiation from Dr. Rounsaville and enthusiastically embraced imagery as a healing practice. Mike imagined the radiation as a golden light that permeated his lungs, melting away any tumor and leaving a golden glow within him. He regarded the radiation machine and the doctors, nurses, and technicians who treated him as angels sent to help him heal. He had active Inner Healers with whom he consulted regularly, and he prayed daily, though his prayers were strictly prayers of gratitude and he never asked for anything for himself. He also took a wide variety of cancer-fighting supplements, though he never changed his diet and didn't quit smoking for several years after his diagnosis. While most people diagnosed at his stage of cancer survive only a year or so, Mike lived six good-quality years past his diagnosis before passing away from heart disease. There was no evidence of cancer in his body.

Sato-Perry says that like most people with cancer, patients going through radiation have issues of power and participation: "I want people to be centered enough to have their own unique experience, not fall into another's suggestion or statistic. That happens best when they can get strong signals from within themselves. I like to see [people going through radiation] wake up to their power in the face of such extraordinary, external power—the hospital, medical staff, the radiation machine with both its size and mystique. But the truth is, that machine has only a fraction of the supreme sophistication of their mind-body-spirit."

If you choose to have radiation, go into it intending for it to work exactly the way you want. Take some time to consult with your Inner Healer about how best to imagine and use the power of the radiation to eliminate cancer cells, and also ask how you can help protect any normal cells in the area at the same time. Use your own imagery as it comes to you in the following imagery script. As always, make use of your Healing Journal, and have writing and drawing implements handy.

Making the Most of Your Radiation Therapy

Take a comfortable position and let yourself begin to relax in your own way . . . let your breathing get a little deeper and fuller . . . but still comfortable . . . with every breath in, notice that you bring in fresh air, fresh oxygen, fresh energy that fuels your body . . . and with every breath out, imagine that you can release a bit of tension . . . a bit of discomfort . . . a bit of worry . . . and let that deeper breathing and the thoughts you have of fresh energy in and tension and worry out be an invitation to your body and mind to begin to relax . . . to begin to shift gears . . . and let it be an easy and natural movement . . . without having to force anything . . . without having to make anything happen right now . . . just letting it happen . . . just breathing and relaxing . . . breathing and energizing. . . .

Come back to taking a few deeper breaths whenever you feel like relaxing even more deeply . . . but for now, let your breathing take its own natural rate and its own natural rhythm . . . and simply let the gentle movement of your body as it breathes allow you to relax naturally and comfortably . . . almost without having to try. . . .

And noticing how your right foot feels right now . . . and how your left foot feels . . . and noticing that just before you probably weren't aware of your feet at all . . . but now that you turn your attention to them, you can notice them and how they feel . . . and notice the intelligence that is there in your feet . . . and notice what happens when you silently invite your feet to relax . . . and become soft and at ease . . . and in the same way noticing the intelligence in your legs and releasing your legs . . . and letting the intelligence in your legs respond in their own way . . . and noticing any release and relaxation that happens . . . without having to make any effort at all . . . just softening and releasing . . . and letting it be a comfortable and very pleasant experience. . . .

And you can relax even more deeply and comfortably if you want to . . . by continuing to notice the intelligence in different parts of your body and inviting them to soften and relax . . . and noticing how they relax . . . and you are in control of your relaxation and only relax as deeply as is comfortable for you . . . and if you ever need to return your awareness to the outer world you can do that by opening your eyes and looking around and coming fully alert . . . and if you need to respond to anything there you can do that . . . and knowing that you can do this if you need to . . . you can relax again and return your attention to the inner world of your imagination. . . .

Inviting the intelligence of your low back, pelvis, and hips to release and relax . . . and your abdomen and midsection . . . and your chest and rib cage . . . without effort or struggle . . . just letting go but staying aware as you do. . . .

Inviting the intelligence in your back and spine to soften and release . . . in your low back . . . mid-back . . . between and across your shoulder blades . . . and across your neck and shoulders . . . the intelligence in your arms . . . and elbows . . . and forearms . . . through your wrists and hands . . . and the palms of the hands . . . the fingers . . . and thumbs. . . .

Noticing the intelligence in your face and jaws and inviting them to relax . . . to become soft and at ease . . . and your scalp and forehead . . . and your eyes . . . even your tongue can be at ease. . . .

And as you relax, let your attention shift from your usual outer world to what we can call your inner world . . . the world inside that only you can see, hear, smell, and feel . . . the world where your memories, your dreams, your feelings, your plans all reside . . . a world that you can learn to connect with . . . that can help you in many ways on your journey. . . .

And imagine that you find inside a very special place . . . a very beautiful place where you feel comfortable and relaxed, yet very aware . . . this may be a place that you have actually visited at some time in your life . . . in the outer world or even in this inner world . . . or it may be a place that you've seen somewhere . . . or it may be a brand-new place that you haven't visited before . . . and none of that matters as long as it is a very beautiful place, a place that invites you and feels good to be in . . . a place that feels safe and healing for you. . . .

And let yourself take some time to explore this place . . . and notice what you imagine seeing there . . . all the things you see . . . and how you see them . . . don't worry at all about how you imagine this place as long as it is beautiful to you and feels safe and healing . . . and notice if there are any sounds you imagine hearing . . . or if it is simply very quiet in your healing place . . . notice if there is a fragrance or aroma that you imagine there or a special quality of the air . . . there may or may not be, and it's perfectly all right however you imagine this place of healing . . . it may change over time as you explore it, or it may stay the same . . . it doesn't matter at this point . . . just let yourself explore a little more. . . .

Can you tell what time of day it is? . . . or what time of year it is? . . . and what the temperature is like? . . . how you are dressed? . . . take some time to find a place where you feel safe and let yourself get comfortable there . . . and just notice how it feels to imagine yourself there . . . and if your mind wanders from time to time, just take another deep breath or two and gently return your attention to this beautiful and healing place . . . just for now . . . without feeling the need to go anywhere else right now . . . or do anything else . . . just for now. . . .

And allow yourself to become aware of anything here that feels healing to you . . . it may be the beauty . . . it may be the sense of peacefulness . . . it may be the temperature, or the fragrance, or a combination of all the qualities that are here . . . perhaps you have a sense of what's sacred to you and what supports you in your life . . . it doesn't matter what you find healing here . . . or whether you can even identify it specifically . . . but let yourself experience whatever healing is there for you . . . and simply relax there . . . and know that while you relax, your body's natural healing systems can operate at their highest efficiency . . . without distraction . . . and without needing to be told what to do. . . .

The same built-in abilities to heal wounds, to repair injuries, to eradicate infections, and to destroy cancer cells that have been with you all your life can now function at full capacity . . . without any diversion of your precious energy . . . so while you relax, your body can take advantage of the time to fuel its ability to heal . . . as your muscles relax, your blood flows in all the right places . . . bringing your immune defenders to every place they are needed . . . and allowing them to efficiently and specifically target any cells that no longer belong to the healthy you . . . engulfing them and removing them . . . to be eliminated whenever you release what's no longer healthy for you . . . with your out breath . . . with your stool and urine . . . even with your sweat . . . and energizing yourself with fresh air and oxygen with every in breath . . . and with nutritious and healthy food . . . and with thoughts that bring you strength, courage, and even joy . . . and just letting yourself rest in this for a while. . . .

As you are enjoying this comfortable state of relaxation, invite an image for any inner support you have to be with you . . . an Inner Healer . . . or images of people that are genuinely support-ive of your healing . . . or of whatever spiritual force supports and guides you . . . and ask for their help in beginning to imagine that the radiation treatment you will receive will work in the very best possible way for you. . . .

Before your treatment begins, focus on any area of your body through which the radiation has to pass to reach the tumor cells . . . imagine in some way that you send love and healing energy to these tissues . . . and ask the healing abilities within you to protect and care for these tissues especially well during your treatment . . . there may be an image that comes to mind for how these cells can be protected and supported during treatment. . . .

You may imagine that the healthy tissues are protected by a shield or protective wrapping, a spiritual force, or a force field or energy that you imagine placing there . . . as if you can wall off and protect any healthy tissues in your body while the radiation kills any cancer cells or tissues . . . or there may be another way that comes to you to imagine this. . . .

And then imagine that the powerful radiation energy can focus and concentrate exactly where it is needed . . . directly in any cancer tissue or tumor . . . killing them rapidly, effectively, and completely . . . you might imagine the radiation as energy rays, as bullets, or any other form of focused lethal energy . . . you might imagine cancer cells or tissues exploding, imploding, melting, shriveling, drying up, or clutching their dark little hearts and dying as the villain always does in movies . . . maybe you have another image and that's even better . . . just imagine the radiation doing what it's meant to do, destroying cancer . . . imagine that happening anyway you imagine it . . . but do it thoroughly . . . and completely . . . imagine it working exactly as you'd like it to—concentrating on eradicating cancer . . . and leaving the healthy cells alone. . . .

Next, after the radiation has killed all the cancer cells in the area, you can imagine a vigorous and aggressive response from your immune defense system . . . imagine billions and billions of immune cells, killer cells, swarming into the area and wiping up any remaining cancer cells, any debris, and chemical residue of the battle and reestablishing a healthy, controlled, well-organized environment into which healthy cells can once again grow . . . they clean up the neighborhood and make it safe once again for good health . . . imagine that there are many hundreds of thousands as many immune cells as cancer cells (because there are), and that they can now easily identify and overcome any remaining cells . . . imagine the cancer cells dead, weak, badly injured, and dazed . . . disorganized and completely vulnerable to the aggressive and highly motivated immune cells . . . and because they are damaged, they leak and give off chemical signals that actually attract killer cells . . . they can no longer hide from them. . . .

Give your immune defense system a cheer and let them know how much you are behind them . . . root them on! . . . maybe there's a cavalry charge sounding in the background . . . maybe there's some other music or some battle cry that they have . . . imagine that they are efficient, aggressive, and without hesitation remove any cells that are not functioning in healthy cooperation with their neighbors and their function in the whole person . . . pour it on . . . a lot of energy goes into this . . . and imagine that your immune system will remain strong and powerful throughout . . . on the job twenty-four hours a day . . . waking or sleeping . . . and that every time you check in on them and support them this way it encourages them to fight on. . . .

Take some time to notice what it feels like to have these powerful combined forces on your side. . . .

Now imagine that you move into the future . . . sometime in the not too distant future when your radiation treatment is all over and you have had the very best outcome you can imagine . . . and that you are once again doing the things that you enjoy . . . with the people you love to do them with . . . and enjoying a restored sense of good health . . . imagine that you are feeling very good about making the best use of your treatment and getting the very best results from it . . . having the treatment work just the way that you imagine it working . . . and feeling very good about it.

And imagine yourself year after year, perhaps with one of those calendars where the pages fly off the wall, visiting your doctor from time to time and your doctor examining your tests, your body, and smiling, giving you good news . . . both you and your doctors feeling very, very good about the successful treatment you have received . . . and seeing yourself as far into the future as you'd like to imagine yourself, doing things that are meaningful and enjoyable to you . . . and feeling very grateful that you are able to get good treatment and make the very best use of it. . . .

Taking all the time you need. . . .

And when you are ready to return your attention to the outer world, silently express any appreciation you might have for having a special healing place within you . . . and for being able to use your imagination in this way . . . and for the healing capabilities that have been built into you by nature . . . and for the radiation and other treatments that are helping you fight cancer . . . and when you are ready, allow all the images to fade and go back within . . . knowing that healing continues to happen within you at all times . . . and gently bring your attention back to the room around you and the current time and place . . . and bring back with you anything that seems important or interesting to bring back, including any feelings of comfort, relaxation, or healing . . . and when you are all the way back, gently stretch and open your eyes. . . .

And take a few minutes to write or draw about your experience.

Debriefing Your Experience

As usual, write or draw what seemed significant or interesting to you about this experience. Following that, answer the following, if you haven't already:

How do you feel after doing this process?
How did you imagine protecting your healthy cells?
How might you in the future?
How did you imagine the radiation?
How did you imagine directing radiation to the cancer cells, and how did they react when radiation came in contact with them?
How might you imagine the radiation being even more powerful in the future?
How did you imagine your immune response?
How might that be imagined even more powerfully in the future?
How did you imagine yourself in the future?
How did you look?
How far in the future was this?
What were you doing?
Who were you with?
Are there other future images that would also bring positive motivation to you?

What seemed most important or interesting to you about your imagery this time?

Making the Most of Nutrition, Healing, and Other Treatments

You can, and probably should, include everything you do for yourself in your imagery of healing. On top of your chemotherapy, radiation, and/or surgery, consider nutrition. If you've changed your diet in order to support your healing abilities, include that in your imagery. Just think about the healing power of that carrot, broccoli, vitamin C, those Chinese herbs, or whatever you choose to eat. Once you decide to eat something, imagine that it's good for you. Maybe there's a chemical benefit in the emotional satisfaction gained from that piece of chocolate that more than counterbalances the potential effects of refined sugar. Don't be afraid to eat what feels right to you, but bless it as you eat it, consecrate it, and find a way to bring it inside with the affirmation that it is dedicated to healing.

If you feel you're fooling yourself with this approach, then consider making other food choices. Ask yourself why you'd make a choice that wasn't supportive of healing. The purpose is not to blame yourself but to stay clear on what your intention is, and how you imagine you can make that intention a reality.

Every acupuncture treatment, every massage, every talk with a friend, every walk, breath, prayer, or thought you have can be dedicated or blessed. Imagine that it all supports you, and when you notice things that do not, then begin to think about how you could change those situations, or accept them if you feel they cannot be changed.

There are only two reasons I know of to do any medical or healing treatment: it makes you feel better or it has the potential to extend your life. Whatever you choose to use to support your health, approach it as if it will work. Do it so that if it's up to you, the outcome will be the one you want.

In the movie *Little Big Man*, Dustin Hoffman plays a young man who has been brought up part white, part Indian (Native American). His Indian "grandfather" is a classic chief, dripping with dignity and wisdom in all that he says and does. One day he decides it is his day to die. He packs his blanket, his medicine bag, and sings his death song to the Great Spirit. He ceremonially lies down on his blanket, closes his eyes, and waits. After hours or days of waiting, he gets up, folds up his blanket, and says to Hoffman, matter-of-factly, "Sometimes the magic works and sometimes it doesn't."

We usually do not know in advance what we can do and what we can't. Henry Ford said, "Whether you think you can or you can't, you're probably right." Always do your healing work as if it will work and as if it is up to you. If it is, you will heal. If it isn't, you might heal anyway.

Summary

+ Guided imagery is useful in reducing undesired effects from radiation therapy.
+ Incorporate other treatments you employ, from nutrition to complementary treatments, into your imagery and your intention to heal.
+ A specific guided imagery script for radiation will allow you to imagine making the most of this treatment.

10

Relieving Pain

Although pain is not an issue for many people with cancer, it is frequent enough to deserve our attention here. Guided imagery is effective in relieving pain, whether from procedures, post-surgery, or from cancer and is especially effective in relieving the amplification effect that emotions have on pain.

Pain is a complex experience that consists of two major aspects: the physical sensation of a pain nerve being stimulated and our reactions to it. The first element is called nociceptive pain and the second is called suffering. Suffering is an emotional component of pain that can often be its greater part. The areas in the brain that process and transmit pain signals are close to or sometimes identical with the areas that process emotions, and the neurotransmitter chemicals in the brain that signal pain or emotion are closely interrelated. This perhaps explains why fear and other unpleasant emotions can amplify pain, but it also lets us know that there are connections inside that can help reduce or relieve pain.

Many studies have shown that relaxation and guided imagery can significantly relieve pain in cancer patients, whether the pain is postoperative or from some aspect of cancer.[1] Of course, there are other effective ways to control pain, including medications, physical therapy, and acupuncture, but using the pain-relieving powers of your own mind adds a greater sense of control, a greater confidence in the abilities of your own mind to affect your body, and relief from emotional tension that may be compounding and amplifying pain.

I have often seen imagery and nonpharmacological methods work to relieve serious pain, even pain that could not be relieved with medications. It is when pain cannot be relieved by medications that imagery may work best, because it can address the mental and emotional components that medications do not.

Mary was a seventy-four-year-old grandmother who had Stage 4 lung cancer and severe chest pain. No medications had been able to relieve her pain and she was referred to me. In the process of asking her about her pain I also asked her about her life. She told me about many things—her children and grandchildren, the sorrow she was feeling about imminently leaving them, and finally about her troubled and abusive marriage. She cried as she related how cruel her husband had been to her, and what a relief it would be to finally be safe from him. After a while she composed herself and thanked me for listening to her. She said it was the first time she had ever told anybody about how she was actually feeling. I then asked how she felt about telling me, and she said, "Very relieved. And, I can't believe it, but my chest pain is gone!"

This isn't to say that anyone's pain is all emotional, but emotional pain is real, and many people feel it physically. It can also dramatically amplify pain from physical causes and make it intolerable.

The distance between how you want things to be and how things are is called suffering. Its resolution depends, therefore, on reducing or eliminating that distance, one way or the other. One way is changing the way things are, and the other way is to change how you perceive things to be.

Imagery has powerful physiological consequences that are directly related to the healing systems of the body. Research on the omnipresent placebo effect, the standard to which we compare all other modalities (and find relatively few more powerful), has provided some of the strongest evidence for the power of the imagination and positive faith in healing. It is well documented that from 30 to 55 percent of all patients given inactive placebos respond as well or better than those given active treatments or agents.[2]

This pain-relieving placebo effect, which as we have previously discussed could easily be called the healing effect, has been shown to be due to the secretion of endorphins, brain chemicals that are powerful pain relievers. In 1978, researcher Jon Levine, M.D., and his colleagues at UCSF investigated pain in patients after dental procedures. They were able to identify patients who were "placebo responders" by the relief of pain they got after receiving an inactive injection and found that if they then gave these patients a medication that blocked the effects of opiates, they developed pain again. In other words, when patients believed they were getting pain medications, their brains secreted powerful endorphins that relieved their pain.

Endorphins are similar to morphine, and your brain can produce pain-relieving chemicals called dynorphins that are thousands of times more potent. UCLA assistant professor of anesthesiology David Bresler likes to say that the brain is the world's greatest pharmacy and imagery is the key that unlocks it.

Below is a simple imagery process that takes advantage of that capability. This first imagery process includes relaxation, to reduce any muscle tension that can amplify pain. It also uses several imagery techniques aimed at relieving pain directly. Later in this chapter I will teach you an imagery dialogue technique that addresses the emotional aspects of pain. You may find that both have their place, or that one works better than the other. Try them both and use what works best for you.

Before beginning this process, make sure you will not be disturbed for about twenty-five minutes. Have your Healing Journal with you and take a few minutes to describe the nature and intensity of your pain before the imagery experience.

Where is your pain located?

What size and shape does it have?

What qualities does it have?

How intense is it on a scale of 0 to 10, where 0 is no pain, and 10 is the worst you can imagine?

How do you feel in relation to the pain?

What measures have you already tried to relieve the pain and how have they worked?

Now get as comfortable as you can and remember that you can shift or move anytime to be even more comfortable. Go along with the imagery in your own way and let's see how comfortable you can get.

Endorphin Drip Imagery

Take a comfortable position and let yourself begin to relax in your own way . . . let your breathing get a little deeper and fuller . . . but still comfortable . . . with every breath in, notice that you bring in fresh air, fresh oxygen, fresh energy that fuels your body . . . and with every breath out, imagine that you can release a bit of tension . . . a bit of discomfort . . . a bit of worry . . . and let that deeper breathing and the thoughts you have of fresh energy in and tension and worry out be an invitation to your body and mind to begin to relax . . . to begin to shift gears . . . and let it be an easy and natural movement . . . without having to force anything . . . without having to make anything happen right now . . . just letting it happen . . . just breathing and relaxing . . . breathing and energizing. . . .

Come back to taking a few deeper breaths whenever you feel like relaxing even more deeply . . . but for now, let your breathing take its own natural rate and its own natural rhythm . . . and simply let the gentle movement of your body as it breathes allow you to relax naturally and comfortably . . . almost without having to try. . . .

And noticing how your right foot feels right now . . . and how your left foot feels . . . and noticing that just before you probably weren't aware of your feet at all . . . but now that you turn your attention to them, you can notice them and how they feel . . . and notice the intelligence that is there in your feet . . . and notice what happens when you silently invite your feet to relax . . . and become soft and at ease . . . and in the same way noticing the intelligence in your legs and releasing your legs . . . and letting the intelligence in your legs respond in their own way . . . and noticing any release and relaxation that happens . . . without having to make any effort at all . . . just softening and releasing . . . and letting it be a comfortable and very pleasant experience. . . .

And you can relax even more deeply and comfortably if you want to . . . by continuing to notice the intelligence in different parts of your body and inviting them to soften and relax . . . and noticing how they relax . . . and you are in control of your relaxation and only relax as deeply as is comfortable for you . . . and if you ever need to return your awareness to the outer world you can do that by opening your eyes and looking around and coming fully alert . . . and if you need to respond to anything there you can do that . . . and knowing that you can do this if you need to . . . you can relax again and return your attention to the inner world of your imagination. . . .

Inviting the intelligence of your low back, pelvis, and hips to release and relax . . . and your abdomen and midsection . . . and your chest and rib cage . . . without effort or struggle . . . just letting go but staying aware as you do. . . .

Inviting the intelligence in your back and spine to soften and release . . . in your low back . . . mid-back . . . between and across your shoulder blades . . . and across your neck and shoulders . . . the intelligence in your arms . . . and elbows . . . and forearms . . . through your wrists and hands . . . and the palms of the hands . . . the fingers . . . and thumbs. . . .

Noticing the intelligence in your face and jaws and inviting them to relax . . . to become soft and at ease . . . and your scalp and forehead . . . and your eyes . . . even your tongue can be at ease. . . .

And as you relax, let your attention shift from your usual outer world to what we can call your inner world . . . the world inside that only you can see, hear, smell, and feel . . . the world where your memories, your dreams, your feelings, your plans all reside . . . a world that you can learn to connect with . . . that can help you in many ways on your journey. . . .

And imagine that you find inside a very special place . . . a very beautiful place where you feel comfortable and relaxed, yet very aware . . . this may be a place that you have actually visited at some time in your life . . . in the outer world or even in this inner world . . . or it may be a place that you've seen somewhere . . . or it may be a brand-new place that you haven't visited before . . . and none of that matters as long as it is a very beautiful place, a place that invites you and feels good to be in . . . a place that feels safe and healing for you. . . .

And let yourself take some time to explore this place . . . and notice what you imagine seeing there . . . all the things you see . . . and how you see them . . . don't worry at all about how you imagine this place as long as it is beautiful to you and feels safe and healing . . . and notice if there are any sounds you imagine hearing . . . or if it is simply very quiet in your healing place . . . notice if there is a fragrance or aroma that you imagine there or a special quality of the air . . . there may or may not be, and it's perfectly all right however you imagine this place of healing . . . it may change over time as you explore it, or it may stay the same . . . it doesn't matter at this point . . . just let yourself explore a little more. . . .

Can you tell what time of day it is? . . . or what time of year it is? . . . and what the temperature is like? . . . how you are dressed? . . . take some time to find a place where you feel safe and let yourself get comfortable there . . . and just notice how it feels to imagine yourself there . . . and if your mind wanders from time to time, just take another deep breath or two and gently return your attention to this beautiful and healing place . . . just for now . . . without feeling the need to go anywhere else right now . . . or do anything else . . . just for now. . . .

And once again allow yourself to become aware of anything here that feels healing to you . . . it may be the beauty . . . it may be the sense of peacefulness . . . it may be the temperature, or the fragrance, or a combination of all the qualities that are here . . . perhaps you have a sense of what's sacred to you and what supports you in your life . . . it doesn't matter what you find healing here . . . or whether you can even identify it specifically . . . but let yourself experience whatever healing is there for you . . . and simply relax there . . . and know that while you relax, your body's natural healing systems can operate at their highest efficiency . . . without distraction . . . and without needing to be told what to do. . . .

The same built-in abilities to heal wounds, to repair injuries, to eradicate infections, and to destroy cancer cells that have been with you all your life can now function at full capacity . . . without any diversion of your precious energy . . . so while you relax, your body can take advantage of the time to fuel its ability to become more comfortable and heal . . . as your muscles relax, your blood flows in all the right places . . . washing away any discomfort or pain . . . bringing soothing nutrients and repair into any area. . . .

And as you become more and more relaxed . . . focus on any area in your body where you still feel any discomfort . . . and without trying to do anything about it for now, simply observe it for a few moments . . . how intense is the pain on a scale of zero to ten, where ten is the worst? . . . if the pain had a shape, what shape would it be? . . . and how big would it be? . . . if it held water, how much water would it hold? . . . a cup? . . . a quart? . . . a tablespoon? . . . just notice . . . and if it had a color, what color would it be? . . . and just let your breathe come gently in and out of the area for a while . . . and imagine that the area gently expands and shrinks a bit with your breath . . . and now take four deeper breaths and imagine that you breathe directly into the area, and as you breathe out some of the color goes out with the breath . . . breathing comfortably but a little deeper. . . .

And after four breaths let your breathing become automatic again and tune back in to the area again . . . notice how it feels now . . . does it feel the same or different in any way? . . . how big is it now? . . . how much water would it hold now? . . . how intense is it on a scale of zero to ten? . . . and what color is it now? . . .

Imagine that every breath brings more comfort to the area. . . .

And along with the relaxation and blood flow the body can bring powerful chemicals from the brain that can relieve discomfort or pain . . . and you can now focus your attention on a spot in the middle of your head . . . at the bottom and center of your brain . . . just behind the midpoint between your eyes . . . and there is a gland there shaped like a teardrop . . . your pituitary gland . . . and it hangs suspended below the brain, immersed and bathed in a rich flow of your blood . . . and this gland produces powerful chemicals that are the most powerful pain relievers known to man . . . some of these natural brain chemicals are a thousand times stronger than morphine . . . so powerful that a few drops can make you feel comfortable, relaxed and free of pain for hours at a time . . . and you can imagine that a drop full of these powerful pain relievers forms on the bottom of this pituitary gland like a drop of water beading on a faucet . . . and as the drop becomes heavier and heavier with a rich mixture of pain relievers it finally drops off and dissolves into the blood flowing through . . . and the blood, pumped along by the steady beat of your heart, flows down from the brain through your blood vessels . . . and as it flows through the blood vessels that go to every part of your body, the chemicals attach to receptor sites in the tissues like keys in a lock . . . and they tell the tissues to turn off any pain signals and become calm and comfortable . . . and as that happens you can allow yourself to go deeper and deeper into a state of deep comfort and relaxation . . . and you can adjust and continue the drip of pain relievers into your bloodstream so that they saturate the tissues of your body, especially in the area where you have been experiencing pain or discomfort . . . and as they saturate the area, the area becomes more and more comfortable. . . .

And now imagine that you are comfortably lying on your back watching a single fluffy cloud floating through a clear blue sky . . . that you see it come in one side of your vision and just lazily watch it slowly drift along . . . with nothing else to do . . . and nowhere else to go . . . and noticing the shapes it takes as it slowly drifts by. . . .

And as it starts to float over your head, imagine that it slowly begins to take on the color of any discomfort you have left . . . slowly changing as if it is drawing the discomfort out of your body and into itself . . . and its shape slowly changes to be the exact shape of the discomfort . . . and the color . . . and it absorbs as much as it can . . . and continues to float along . . . slowly . . . drifting away from you now . . . and you can continue to watch it with curiosity . . . as it drifts farther and farther away . . . and keep watching it until you can barely see it . . . until you can't quite tell whether you can see it or not. . . .

And if there is still any discomfort . . . another fluffy white cloud can drift into view . . . and take on its shape and color . . . and drift slowly out of sight . . . until you can't really tell whether it is there or not . . . and you can watch these clouds drift by and feel more comfortable as long as you like. . . .

Taking all the time you need. . . .

And when you are ready to return your attention to the outer world, silently express any appreciation you might have for having a special healing place within you . . . and for being able to use your imagination in this way . . . and for the healing capabilities that have been built into you by nature. . . .

And when you are ready, allow all the images to fade and go back within . . . knowing that healing continues to happen within you at all times . . . and gently bring your attention back to the room around you and the current time and place . . . and bring back with you anything that seems important or interesting to bring back, including any feelings of comfort, relaxation, or healing . . . and when you are all the way back, gently stretch and open your eyes. . . .

And take a few minutes to write or draw about your experience.

Debriefing Your Experience

As usual, take some time to write or draw in your Healing Journal. If you haven't already, consider the following questions about your experience.

How do you feel after doing this process?

How is your comfort or discomfort level now?

Is it the same or different?

How intense is your discomfort on a 1-to-10 scale?

How does that compare to when you started?

What qualities does any discomfort have now?

Are these the same or different than before?

How do you feel about the pain and your relationship to it now?

Do you feel the same or different?

What seemed most interesting or important to you about this process?

What aspects seemed most effective to you?

How will you use this process in the future?

If you had some success with this first effort, it is a very positive sign, and I would encourage you to use this process frequently since it will have a cumulative effect. If you did not experience pain relief the first time, try the next process, and then use one or the other at least six times to see if either helps you.

The Dialogue with Pain

This next imagery process is a powerful way of exploring the meaning and emotional aspects of pain and of negotiating pain reduction or relief. It makes use of the same imagery dialogue technique you use when communicating with your Inner Healer, but here you'll address your pain directly by inviting an image to come to mind and exploring why the pain is there and what it will take to get it to go away.

It may seem strange to want to communicate with pain, but pain is a signal from your body. Like the oil light on your car, pain signals you that something needs attention, and, like the oil light, it might be a mistake to eliminate it without knowing what needs attention.

Just because you are fighting cancer doesn't mean that the pain you experience is from cancer—you can have pain from other areas, just like anyone else. In addition, you may even be more vulnerable to feeling pain intensity because you may be fatigued from treatments and the ongoing psychological stress, even if you are coping well. So "tuning in" to see what your body is trying to tell you makes a lot of sense. At worst, you will be no worse off, and at best you will learn something useful in your healing and be relieved of pain as well.

This script is especially useful for uncovering and resolving the emotional meaning of pain, and relieving the suffering associated with pain. It is consistently surprising to see how much relief people can get by going through this process, even if there is a clear physical reason for the pain. I encourage you to do an open-minded exploration of this process even if you feel that there is no emotional component to your pain. It is often helpful even if there isn't one. Just try it and then use whichever of the two methods in this chapter that works best for you.

The Dialogue with Pain

Take a comfortable position and let yourself begin to relax in your own way . . . let your breathing get a little deeper and fuller . . . but still comfortable . . . with every breath in, notice that you bring in fresh air, fresh oxygen, fresh energy that fuels your body . . . and with every breath out, imagine that you can release a bit of tension . . . a bit of discomfort . . . a bit of worry . . . and let that deeper breathing and the thoughts you have of fresh energy in and tension and worry out be an invitation to your body and mind to begin to relax . . . to begin to shift gears . . . and let it be an easy and natural movement . . . without having to force anything . . . without having to make anything happen right

now . . . just letting it happen . . . just breathing and relaxing . . . breathing and energizing. . . .

Come back to taking a few deeper breaths whenever you feel like relaxing even more deeply . . . but for now, let your breathing take its own natural rate and its own natural rhythm . . . and simply let the gentle movement of your body as it breathes allow you to relax naturally and comfortably . . . almost without having to try. . . .

And noticing how your right foot feels right now . . . and how your left foot feels . . . and noticing that just before you probably weren't aware of your feet at all . . . but now that you turn your attention to them, you can notice them and how they feel . . . and notice the intelligence that is there in your feet . . . and notice what happens when you silently invite your feet to relax . . . and become soft and at ease . . . and in the same way noticing the intelligence in your legs and releasing your legs . . . and letting the intelligence in your legs respond in their own way . . . and noticing any release and relaxation that happens . . . without having to make any effort at all . . . just softening and releasing . . . and letting it be a comfortable and very pleasant experience. . . .

And you can relax even more deeply and comfortably if you want to . . . by continuing to notice the intelligence in different parts of your body and inviting them to soften and relax . . . and noticing how they relax . . . and you are in control of your relaxation and only relax as deeply as is comfortable for you . . . and if you ever need to return your awareness to the outer world you can do that by opening your eyes and looking around and coming fully alert . . . and if you need to respond to anything there you can do that . . . and knowing that you can do this if you need to . . . you can relax again and return your attention to the inner world of your imagination. . . .

Inviting the intelligence of your low back, pelvis, and hips to release and relax . . . and your abdomen and midsection . . . and your chest and rib cage . . . without effort or struggle . . . just letting go but staying aware as you do. . . .

Inviting the intelligence in your back and spine to soften and release . . . in your low back . . . mid-back . . . between and across your shoulder blades . . . and across your neck and shoulders . . . the intelligence in your arms . . . and elbows . . . and forearms . . . through your wrists and hands . . . and the palms of the hands . . . the fingers . . . and thumbs. . . .

Noticing the intelligence in your face and jaws and inviting them to relax . . . to become soft and at ease . . . and your scalp and forehead . . . and your eyes . . . even your tongue can be at ease. . . .

And as you relax, let your attention shift from your usual outer world to what we can call your inner world . . . the world inside that only you can see, hear, smell, and feel . . . the world where your memories, your dreams, your feelings, your plans all reside . . . a world that you can learn to connect with . . . that can help you in many ways on your journey. . . .

And imagine that you find inside a very special place . . . a very beautiful place where you feel comfortable and relaxed, yet very aware . . . this may be a place that you have actually visited at some time in your life . . . in the outer world or even in this inner world . . . or it may be a place that you've seen somewhere . . . or it may be a brand-new place that you haven't visited before . . . and none of that matters as long as it is a very beautiful place, a place that invites you and feels good to be in . . . a place that feels safe and healing for you. . . .

And let yourself take some time to explore this place . . . and notice what you imagine seeing there . . . all the things you see . . . and how you see them . . . don't worry at all about how you imagine this place as long as it is beautiful to you and feels safe and healing . . . and notice if there are any sounds you imagine hearing . . . or if it is simply very quiet in your healing place . . . notice if there is a fragrance or aroma that you imagine there or a special quality of the air . . . there may or may not be, and it's perfectly all right however you imagine this place of healing . . . it may change over time as you explore it, or it may stay the same . . . it doesn't matter at this point . . . just let yourself explore a little more. . . .

Can you tell what time of day it is? . . . or what time of year it is? . . . and what the temperature is like? . . . how you are dressed? . . . take some time to find a place where you feel safe and let yourself get comfortable there . . . and just notice how it feels to imagine yourself there . . . and if your mind wanders from time to time, just take another deep breath or two and gently return your attention to this beautiful and healing place . . . just for now . . . without feeling the need to go anywhere else right now . . . or do anything else . . . just for now. . . .

And once again allow yourself to become aware of anything here that feels healing to you . . . it may be the beauty . . . it may be the sense of peacefulness . . . it may be the temperature, or the fragrance, or a combination of all the qualities that are here . . . perhaps you have a sense of what's sacred to you and what supports you in your life . . . it doesn't matter what you find healing here . . . or whether you can even identify it specifically . . . but let yourself experience whatever healing is there for you . . . and simply relax there . . . and know that while you relax, your body's natural healing systems can operate at their highest efficiency . . . without distraction . . . and without needing to be told what to do. . . .

And as you relax in this special place, you may want to invite your Inner Healer to be there with you . . . lending its presence and healing qualities to your inquiry . . . and welcome your Inner Healer . . . and thank it for being there in whatever form it has come. . . .

And when you are ready, focus on any pain that you have and want to know more about . . . just let your attention come to rest on it without trying to do anything about it for now . . . and letting it know that you are here to understand if there is anything it wants you to know, allow an image to form that can represent this pain . . . and simply allow the image to come to mind . . . and allow it to be whatever it is for now . . . whether it is something you recognize or understand or not . . . it may be something familiar to you or something new . . . just let it be whatever it is and take some time to carefully observe the image . . . how does it look? . . . how big is it? . . . and how big is it in relation to you? . . . what features do you notice especially? . . . observe it from any angle and any distance that is comfortable for you . . . without trying to change it for now . . . just observing . . . what is it doing, if anything? . . .

What qualities does the image seem to embody? . . . name all the qualities you sense in it . . . and how do you feel in its presence? . . . notice all the feelings you have about it or toward it . . . and let them be there . . . are there any other feelings you have toward or about it?. . . .

And when you are ready, thank the image for coming . . . and notice how it responds . . . tell the image how you feel about and toward it . . . in your mind, tell it honestly and directly about all the feelings it brings up . . . and let it respond to that . . . and imagine that it can communicate with you in a way you can understand . . . whether it talks . . . or changes forms . . . or you simply understand it directly. . . .

Ask it if it has anything to tell you that's important for you to know . . . and let it answer for itself . . . and listen carefully to its response . . . and ask it how that's connected to your pain . . . and listen carefully to what it tells you. . . .

And ask it what it wants from you . . . and listen to what it says . . . just listen . . . without judging or arguing right now . . . ask it what it needs from you, and let it respond . . . and ask it if it's trying to do something for you . . . and let it answer . . . and what would it take for it to become less intense or even go away? . . . let it tell or show you. . . .

Consider what you've learned from the image . . . consider what it needs and what it will take for it to go away . . . is this something you are willing and able to give it? . . . if so, is it something internal that you can do right now, or is it something you must do in the outer world? . . .

Is there any obstacle to you giving it what it wants and needs? . . . if so, how might you work out an agreement with it? . . . let it know what's in the way and see if you can negotiate an agreement with it. . . .

Ask it if it would be willing to reduce your pain right now so you can see that it really has the power to do this—even temporarily . . . if it's willing, notice what happens to your pain . . . and if it's not, ask it what it would take for a demonstration of its ability to take away your pain . . . and see if you can reach an agreement that works for both of you. . . .

If you make an agreement with the image, make sure it's one that you will do your best to keep . . . if you're not fully certain, then make arrangements with the image to continue the dialogue until you can find a good agreement for both sides . . . you might ask your Inner Healer for help if you reach an impasse . . . and see what it has to add. . . .

And if you've reached an agreement that can be completed internally, do that now . . . do your part and notice how the image carries out its part . . . and if there's an external component to the agreement, imagine yourself carrying this out with integrity. . . .

And thank the image for coming . . . observe it once again . . . is it the same or different in any way? . . . what have you learned from it? . . . how do you feel toward it now? . . . express anything you appreciate to it . . . and make any arrangements to get back together with it later if there's more to discuss. . . .

And thank your Inner Healer as well . . . and take a minute to review what has happened in this experience . . . and especially notice anything you want to make sure to remember when you come back to waking. . . .

Taking all the time you need. . . .

And when you are ready to return your attention to the outer world, silently express any appreciation you might have for having a special healing place within you . . . and for being able to use your imagination in this way . . . and for the healing capabilities that have been built into you by nature. . . .

And when you are ready, allow all the images to fade and go back within . . . knowing that healing continues to happen within you at all times . . . and gently bring your attention back to the room around you and the current time and place . . . and bring back with you anything that seems important or interesting to bring back, including any feelings of comfort, relaxation, or healing . . . and when you are all the way back, gently stretch and open your eyes. . . .

And take a few minutes to write or draw about your experience.

Debriefing Your Experience

As usual, take some time to write or draw in your Healing Journal. If you haven't already, consider the following questions about your experience.

How do you feel after doing this process?
How is your comfort/discomfort level now?
Is it the same or different?
How intense is your discomfort on a 1-to-10 scale?
How does that compare to when you started?
What qualities does any discomfort have now?
Are these the same or different than before?
What was the image of your pain? (You may want to draw it.)
What did it want and need from you?
What was it trying to do for you?
Did you reach an agreement with it?
If so, what is your end of the bargain?
And what did it say it would do?
Were you able to complete your bargain internally or do you need to do something externally?
If so, when and how will you carry this out?
How do you feel about the pain and your relationship to it now?
Do you feel the same or different?
What seemed most interesting or important to you about this process?
How will you use this process in the future?

Both these pain relief processes can and should be used as often as needed. But if you use the dialogue with pain, keep your bargains or renegotiate in good faith. You are building an internal relationship and improving your mind-body relationship by opening these lines of communication. Treat this with the respect you would any other relationship. If you forget your agreements or renege, you may breed more distrust between your mind and your body—just the opposite of what you are trying to do. If something comes up, go inside and invite the image back into your awareness and ask it if it would be willing to renegotiate. If it is, do it in good faith. There is nobody to fool but you.

In the next chapter we'll address some aspects of spirituality that can be important in healing, and explore a bigger perspective on your life that can illuminate your healing path.

Summary

+ Not all people with cancer have pain, but it may accompany surgery, medical procedures, tumor effects, or come from other causes.
+ Not all pain in people with cancer is actually from cancer, so it needs to be well diagnosed.
+ Pain is both a physical sensation and an emotional experience. The way you manage stress, tension, and emotions can amplify or reduce pain.
+ Pain, depending on its source, can be relieved with medications, physical therapy, and acupuncture, along with guided imagery.
+ Pain can be a valuable guide to what needs attention, and pain relief can come from paying attention to it in the right way.
+ Guided imagery can be helpful with both the physical and emotional aspects of pain control.

11

Spiritual Aspects
of Cancer and Healing

Getting cancer can become the beginning
of living. The search for one's own being, the
discovery of the life one needs to live, can be one
of the strongest weapons against disease.
—*Lawrence LeShan*, You Can Fight for Your Life

If you are lucky enough to have a firm and unshakable belief in something larger and more powerful than you, something that can be trusted no matter what, and that faith is unshaken even by your cancer diagnosis, then you have a tremendous resource of strength on which to draw. A good deal of research shows that a strong spiritual belief system has many advantages for health and well-being. Drs. Elizabeth Targ and Ellen Levine, researchers at California Pacific Medical Center in San Francisco, studied women with early breast cancer and characterized their health, functional well-being, and spiritual belief systems. They found a strong correlation between a strong belief system and functional well-being, including physical health measures.[1] Because many people with strong spiritual beliefs tend to congregate with others who have similar beliefs, the researchers separated the effects of the social support from the belief in something larger and found that the spiritual belief itself was nearly twice as powerful as the accompanying social support.

In addition to your beliefs, quite a few studies show that prayer has a positive influence on health and well-being. Praying can of course bring you comfort and peace of mind but some studies indicate that others praying for your health, whether they are close or far, and whether you know them or not, also can have an influence. In 1988 Robert Byrd reported in the *Southern Journal of Medicine* that people recovering from heart attacks in the coronary care unit of a hospital belonging to the University of California San Francisco recovered better if they were being prayed for—even though they were being prayed for from a distance, by people they didn't know, and the patients didn't know anyone was praying for them. These patients were released in less time, had fewer complications and better coronary function than patients for whom nobody was praying.[2] This study, controversial as it has been, has now been replicated more than once, and was most recently validated by a study published in the *Archives of Internal Medicine*.[3]

Another study, by psychiatrist Elizabeth Targ, reported that HIV patients prayed for by strangers, at a distance, had improved immune system measures and better clinical outcomes than a randomized control group who were not the focus of prayer.[4] This study is extremely well designed and if replicated will provide strong evidence for this effect for those who need the proof.

If you can pray for someone you don't know thousands of miles away and have a positive effect on their health, it makes it a lot easier to imagine that you could affect your own health in the same way.

Imagery and Prayer

The only difference between imagery and prayer in my opinion is who you think you're talking to. If you think you're using your brain to influence your body, it's imagery. If you think it's asking a power greater than you for help, it's prayer. Imagery is great for people who don't have a strong or well-formed spiritual belief system or who don't think God is a humanlike entity they can directly address. It's also great for people who are physiologically based in their thinking, since we know so many neural, endocrine, and immune pathways that imagery can work through. But if you do believe in prayer, imagery can also be a powerful way to pray. The Bible says that God helps those who help themselves, so you might think of your imagery both as a self-help method *and* a prayer. If you believe in God, by whatever name, and it is acceptable to your beliefs, address that being as a source of life and health and ask that your images become manifest and for help to pray even more effectively.

There are many forms of prayer. There are prayers of thanksgiving, where we express our appreciation for the gifts we have been given. There are prayers where we praise the power that created us. There are prayers for help, where we ask for healing, or for specific aid for ourselves or others, and there are prayers that we be made aware of God's will and be of assistance. There are prayers written in every religion, culture, and language that may be especially meaningful to you, and there are the prayers that well up in our hearts when we are in deep contemplation or fear and addressing God directly. However you pray, your imagery may add another dimension, or, conversely, your prayer may consecrate and bless your imagery.

If you have been turned off by religious distortions of spirituality or if your beliefs are not certain, opportunities as well as challenges can arise from having cancer. One of these is the opportunity to clarify what you really believe to be true about yourself, your relationships, and your relationship to life. The fear and uncertainty that so often vividly accompany cancer also seem to be fertile ground for bringing to mind our beliefs about where life comes from, where it goes after death, and what it means while we are here. The imagery methods I offer in this book are compatible with virtually every way I know of worshiping God, a higher power, life, or whatever your belief calls the mystery that underlies all.

Although cancer is by no means a death sentence, it often brings thoughts of death and mortality much more into the foreground of our awareness. This is stressful, but it can also be surprisingly vitalizing. It seems that there are few things better than contemplation of our mortality for bringing a certain sense of vitality and appreciativeness to life.

Therapist and minister Wayne Muller, author of the book *How, Then, Shall We Live?*, writes:

> If we buy the illusion that we will live forever, we can waste all the time in the world before we are ready to live. . . . Proximity to death wakes us up . . . to embrace death is not morbid; to deny death is morbid. If we know we will die, then we will know we are alive. From this mindful awareness can spring a variety of practices that deepen and enrich our time on this earth.

The point here is not to accept imminent death simply because you have cancer, but to notice whether the heightened awareness you have of it can be a way to potentially enrich your life and heighten your appreciation of the experiences life brings you. In many premodern cultures, in which people hunt for their food or slaughter their own animals, and in which death from infectious disease, famine, and war may run rampant, death, though still undesirable, is often seen as an ally that reminds us that life in this form is precious precisely because it is limited.

The Gifts of Mortality

In many premodern cultures, death is acknowledged every day and used as a guide to help form a warrior or spiritual consciousness. The existence of death helps us sort out what is truly important, what is of lasting value, and what really deserves our attention. In many traditions this awareness is cultivated as a lifetime practice, not as simply a scary thing to be faced only when it can no longer be ignored.

Death is not addressed in medical training, even though much of medicine is aimed at preventing it. Some psychologists believe that students going into medicine have a greater fear of death than the average person. Whether that is true or not, an exploration of our thoughts about it can deepen our appreciation of the healer's task. The eminent medical educator Rachel Naomi Remen, M.D., created a course for medical students called The Healer's Art, which is now being taught in many medical schools around the country. In the course, difficult issues in medicine are examined, and experienced physicians gather with small groups of students to encourage them to explore their observations, thoughts, and feelings about these things. One of the most moving sessions addresses death and dying. One of the medical students in my small group shared this observation: "Death seems to strip away false fronts and layers of roles that people become attached to. People act differently when people are dying or facing death—they say things they wouldn't ordinarily say and do things they wouldn't ordinarily do." He related a story of how his father, an accomplished, responsible family man who never asked for help, finally came to ask for help in as simple a thing as buttoning his pajamas, because his illness had diminished his capacity to do that. Tears came to this young man's eyes as he spoke of how deeply meaningful that was for him as a son to have his father ask him for help, and he felt his father accepted it as a part of his own spiritual growth. We often see what's real to people when death enters the picture, and maybe that's what is most scary if we have been avoiding doing this for a long time.

In her class, Dr. Remen asks medical students to contemplate the following questions about their perceptions of death to start a process of detoxifying the idea of death. Taking some time to do this may serve you well, whether or not you are in imminent danger of passing from this life. Take some time to reflect on these and write your responses in your Healing Journal. Notice what each question teaches you about your relationship to life.

+ What is your personal definition of death?
+ What do you wonder about regarding death?
+ If you could ask someone who died some questions, what would those questions be?
+ If you could ask the person only one question, what would it be?
+ What do you imagine the person would answer?

An Interesting Perspective on Death

There are many deaths and rebirths in a normal life. The infant dies as the child develops, and the child gives way to the adult. The single self disappears into the marriage and the parent gives way to the grand-parent. Dreams, abilities, relationships, and responsibilities all have life cycles, and letting go of one that is over allows the beginning of a new cycle of learning and growth. Could the physical passing of the body be another cycle?

Dr. Irving Oyle, one of my great mentors, used to ask us to imagine what it would be like to be conscious as a fetus. You are essentially a water-dwelling plant, attached by a stalk to your mother, and all your nutrient needs pass to you through this stalk. It is dark, quiet, warm, and a reassuring heartbeat drums constantly in the background. There is nothing you have to do and nothing changes much from moment to moment, day to day.

One day you start to feel movement in your environment, and an intermittent sensation of pressure, as if the walls are closing in on you. At first you're not sure, because it lets up fairly quickly, and there are long periods of time in between, but then the movement starts to get regular and rhythmic. You can now feel that the space around you is shrinking, and it's getting uncomfortable. You can't move the same way and you don't know what's happening. Suddenly, the water drains from the space around you and the pressure starts to get intense. You feel like something's trying to push you out, you don't want to go, you didn't ask for this, and besides, there doesn't seem to be anywhere to go. Your head is being squeezed and the small opening you might be able to feel is not even close to being large enough to go through. Your blood supply is getting choked off, too, as the pressure gets more intense. You don't know what's happening and you can't imagine surviving it.

Finally, after an agonizingly long time, the pressure eases up and you arrive in a cold, overly bright, noisy, confusing place where someone holds you upside down and slaps you on the bottom, or puts a rubber suction bulb in your nose and mouth. There are loud voices and sounds you never heard before and you have no idea of what's going on. It's scary and uncomfortable and you don't want to be there. Then someone washes you with warm water, wraps you snugly in a warm blanket, and your mother holds you in her arms for the first time. You can faintly hear the beating of her heart again, and you feel safe once more.

The point of this story is that we do not know what happens after death any more than we know what this life is going to be like. If you knew it was going to be all right in advance, would that help you go through the process more easily? The fetus has no way of knowing what birth leads to, and we're in the same position when we think about death.

Mysteries of Meaning

The idea of death bothers most people, but then, in the big picture, we don't really understand how it fits into the larger plan of life. How do we know that our death doesn't motivate someone else to find a new medical cure, or become a spiritual leader, or appreciate life more? Novelist Kurt Vonnegut reminds us: "Consider the life of the yeast cell. All it ever does is eat, eliminate, and reproduce. Eat, eliminate and reproduce. It never knows it's making champagne."

Besides not knowing what death really brings us, we often don't know what cancer may bring us or give to others that surround us. My favorite uncle developed an acute leukemia suddenly at the age of sixty-four. In spite of the fact that as a young man he would faint at the sight of blood, he went bravely through intensive chemotherapy for months, spending a great deal of time in the hospital. An accountant by profession, he had a strong love of art and was a talented amateur painter. While he was isolated in the hospital and feeling depressed and anxious, my brother, a physician, suggested that he might paint to pass the time and occupy his mind. His daughters brought him art materials and he began to do watercolor caricatures of his caretakers and of his hospital room. It lifted his spirits and fascinated the staff, who became unusually fond of him and related well to his impressions and drawings.

At his request I sent him some guided imagery tapes so he could start to imagine his treatments working well. When he began to experience internal imagery, he described it as "different than anything I've ever encountered before." Excited, he began to paint his internal images of healing. It felt good to feel he could do something to contribute to his healing. He did surprisingly well during his aggressive chemotherapy, and his physicians as well as the art therapy department became very interested in what he was doing. Previously they had been using art therapy in cancer treatment only with children.

They realized that my uncle's paintings, and the effect they had on him, could be useful to other adult patients. The art therapy department held a show of his and other patients' art and music created during their struggle with cancer. The painting that represented the center of my uncle's healing imagery became the cover of the brochure, and he was invited to talk about his experience with the entire medical staff in their Grand Rounds.

My uncle's work, along with his attitude of optimism and the lack of adverse effects to his toxic treatments, significantly improved the cancer treatment center at the University of Michigan by making art therapy an integral part of treatment. None of us who loved him would ever wish for him to go through what he went through, and yet we all stood in awe of the good that came of his journey through cancer.

Who knows whether this was part of the greater plan and was some type of metaphysical purpose being fulfilled, or was it simply that something good came out of something bad? In either case, when we look for blessings that come out of even a cancer experience, we often find them, and they can bring us comfort.

Viktor Frankl was a psychiatrist who survived the concentration camps of the Holocaust. In his book, *Man's Search for Meaning*, Frankl relates his observation that the continuing belief in life's meaning and purpose sustained many who somehow survived the starvation, torture, and bleakness of the camps. Frankl's perspective on this is antithetical to the way that many of us think about searching for meaning. "Perhaps," he writes, "it is not so much for us to find meaning in life as to *give* meaning to what life brings us."

The issue is not whether you will live or die—you will do both. The issue is how would you like to live, and what legacy would you like to leave when your time does arrive?

If exploring this is of interest to you, take your Healing Journal and consider the following questions. You may want to relax and center yourself in your healing place and call on your inner support system to be with you as you do this, or simply take some quiet time to reflect on each question. There are no "right" answers. This is a private exploration. Give yourself as much time with each question as you need.

+ What qualities and values have been most important to you through your life?
+ What lessons have you learned that you would like to pass on to those who survive you?
+ What messages would you like to leave them with?
+ What would you like them to remember about you when you are gone?
+ What would you like them to say about you at your funeral?
+ What epitaph would you like to see on your gravestone?
+ What legacy would you like to leave created out of what you already have? (A legacy need not be—and the most valuable ones generally are not—financial and material.)
+ What can you do now to ensure that you leave that legacy and the lessons you most value?

If you'd like to explore these issues further, here's an imagery process that will help you discover some unusual perspectives on your life. You'll be invited to relax and go to your healing place, and invite your Inner Healer or other sources of support into your awareness. Then you'll imagine that you can view your life from the perspective of your soul just before you came into this lifetime, becoming aware of your ambitions, questions, and concerns at that time. You'll review significant events in your life and then consider all of this in relation to where you are now.

This is not an exercise for the terminally ill—it's one that can open your eyes to what's truly important at any stage of your life—so if you choose to do it don't do it with fear or trepidation, do it as a way to clarify your values and focus your mind on what is important to you.

Your Life in Perspective

Take a comfortable position and let yourself begin to relax in your own way . . . let your breathing get a little deeper and fuller . . . but still comfortable . . . with every breath in, notice that you bring in fresh air, fresh oxygen, fresh energy that fuels your body . . . and with every breath out, imagine that you can release a bit of tension . . . a bit of discomfort . . . a bit of worry . . . and let that deeper breathing and the thoughts you have of fresh energy in and tension and worry out be an invitation to your body and mind to begin to relax . . . to begin to shift gears . . . and let it be an easy and natural movement . . . without having to force anything . . . without having to make anything happen right now . . . just letting it happen . . . just breathing and relaxing . . . breathing and energizing. . . .

Come back to taking a few deeper breaths whenever you feel like relaxing even more deeply . . . but for now, let your breathing take its own natural rate and its own natural rhythm . . . and simply let the gentle movement of your body as it breathes allow you to relax naturally and comfortably . . . almost without having to try. . . .

And noticing how your right foot feels right now . . . and how your left foot feels . . . and noticing that just before you probably weren't aware of your feet at all . . . but now that you turn your attention to them, you can notice them and how they feel . . . and notice the intelligence that is there in your feet . . . and notice what happens when you silently invite your feet to relax . . . and become soft and at ease . . . and in the same way noticing the intelligence in your legs and releasing your legs . . . and letting the intelligence in your legs respond in their own way . . . and noticing any release and relaxation that happens . . . without having to make any effort at all . . . just softening and releasing . . . and letting it be a comfortable and very pleasant experience. . . .

And you can relax even more deeply and comfortably if you want to . . . by continuing to notice the intelligence in different parts of your body and inviting them to soften and relax . . . and noticing how they relax . . . and you are in control of your relaxation and only relax as deeply as is comfortable for you . . . and if you ever need to return your awareness to the outer world you can do that by opening your eyes and looking around and coming fully alert . . . and if you need to respond to anything there you can do that . . . and knowing that you can do this if you need to . . . you can relax again and return your attention to the inner world of your imagination. . . .

Inviting the intelligence of your low back, pelvis, and hips to release and relax . . . and your abdomen and midsection . . . and your chest and rib cage . . . without effort or struggle . . . just letting go but staying aware as you do. . . .

Inviting the intelligence in your back and spine to soften and release . . . in your low back . . . mid-back . . . between and across your shoulder blades . . . and across your neck and shoulders . . . the intelligence in your arms . . . and elbows . . . and forearms . . . through your wrists and hands . . . and the palms of the hands . . . the fingers . . . and thumbs. . . .

Noticing the intelligence in your face and jaws and inviting them to relax . . . to become soft and at ease . . . and your scalp and forehead . . . and your eyes . . . even your tongue can be at ease. . . .

And as you relax, let your attention shift from your usual outer world to what we can call your inner world . . . the world inside that only you can see, hear, smell, and feel . . . the world where your memories, your dreams, your feelings, your plans all reside . . . a world that you can learn to connect with . . . that can help you in many ways on your journey. . . .

And imagine that you find inside a very special place . . . a very beautiful place where you feel comfortable and relaxed, yet very aware . . . this may be a place that you have actually visited at some time in your life . . . in the outer world or even in this inner world . . . or it may be a place that you've seen somewhere . . . or it may be a brand-new place that you haven't visited before . . . and none of that matters as long as it is a very beautiful place, a place that invites you and feels good to be in . . . a place that feels safe and healing for you. . . .

And let yourself take some time to explore this place . . . and notice what you imagine seeing there . . . all the things you see . . . and how you see them . . . don't worry at all about how you imagine this place as long as it is beautiful to you and feels safe and healing . . . and notice if there are any sounds you imagine hearing . . . or if it is simply very quiet in your healing place . . . notice if there is a fragrance or aroma that you imagine there or a special quality of the air . . . there may or may not be, and it's perfectly all right however you imagine this place of healing . . . it may change over time as you explore it, or it may stay the same . . . it doesn't matter at this point . . . just let yourself explore a little more. . . .

Can you tell what time of day it is? . . . or what time of year it is? . . . and what the temperature is like? . . . how you are dressed? . . . take some time to find a place where you feel safe and let yourself get comfortable there . . . and just notice how it feels to imagine yourself there . . . and if your mind wanders from time to time, just take another deep breath or two and gently return your attention to this beautiful and healing place . . . just for now . . . without feeling the need to go anywhere else right now . . . or do anything else . . . just for now. . . .

If you like, invite help and support into your Healing Place . . . anybody or anything that loves you and supports you that you'd like to have there . . . and whatever spiritual force or energy you believe in . . . invite its presence to be there with you . . . and notice how you feel in its presence. . . .

And when you are ready, invite your Inner Healer to be with you . . . and imagine that figure is very wise and very powerful . . . and imagine that you can go back in time and witness your life . . . at first, noticing what you did yesterday . . . and then something from last week . . . and letting that go, something from a year ago . . . and let time slip by as you simply observe what comes to mind . . . something from five years ago . . . and something from your twenties. . . .

Let yourself calmly witness what comes to mind as you continue to move backward, now noticing something from your teens . . . and how you were in that situation . . . and now something from childhood . . . and infancy. . . .

Imagine that you can continue to move backward in time and observe yourself in the womb . . . notice how you are there . . .

and then back to the moment of conception as your father's sperm meets your mother's egg. . . .

And imagine that you continue to be conscious as you move back to the time just before you entered the beginning of this life . . . and imagine that you are there with your Inner Healer . . . and you are contemplating coming into this life . . . notice how you feel . . . are you eager? . . . reluctant? . . . curious? . . . scared? . . . how do you feel? . . . and notice what you are thinking about as you contemplate entering this life . . . what hopes do you have? . . . and what concerns you? . . . what qualities are you bringing in with you? . . . and what do you hope to develop? . . .

Imagine you can ask your Inner Healer for advice about this life and imagine that your Healer answers you in a way you can understand . . . what do you ask? . . . and what is the response? . . . see if there's anything that your Inner Healer wants you to remember above all during this life . . . listen carefully to its advice. . . .

Then imagine that you come into being . . . conception occurs . . . you are once again in the womb . . . and time moves forward once again . . . and you are a child . . . remembering some time when you went through something challenging . . . and noticing what brought you through . . . and now a teen . . . and an adult . . . and remembering a significant time . . . and how you came through it . . . and what you learned . . . and now several years ago . . . and noticing the qualities that seem to always be with you . . . and those that you acquire along the way . . . and now imagine that you come into the present moment . . . and being in this moment, considering what you have brought and learned that can be especially helpful to you now. . . .

And noticing whether you have learned something from this experience that can be helpful now in your healing. . . .

And if you like, you can ask your Inner Healer for its guidance now . . . and as you contemplate the future, notice how you feel . . . and what your thoughts are . . . and if there's anything you know that you especially want to remember as you move forward. . . .

Taking all the time you need. . . .

And when you are ready to return your attention to the outer world, silently express any appreciation you might have for having a special healing place within you . . . and for your Inner Healer . . . and for being able to use your imagination in this way . . . and for the healing capabilities that have been built into you by nature . . . and for anything else you feel grateful for. . . .

And take a minute to review what you want to make sure to bring back with you when you return your attention to the outer world. . . .

And when you know that . . . allow all the images to fade and go back within . . . and gently bring your attention back to the room around you and the current time and place . . . and bring back with you anything that seems important or interesting to bring back . . . and when you are all the way back, gently stretch and open your eyes. . . .

And take a few minutes to write or draw about your experience.

Debriefing Your Experience

As usual, write or draw what seemed significant or interesting to you about this experience. Then answer the following questions, if you haven't already:

How do you feel after doing this?

What did you notice as you imagined moving backwards in time?

How did you perceive yourself in the time before you were born?

What was that experience like?

What were your hopes for this life? Your fears or concerns?

What did you ask your Inner Healer?

How did it respond?

What did your Inner Healer want you to remember above all?

What did you notice as you came into this life and moved forward?

What did you learn that is important as you anticipate moving forward again in your life now?

Summary

+ A strong spiritual belief system is helpful when fighting cancer.
+ In scientific studies prayers have been proven to improve the well-being of cancer patients.
+ Imagery and prayer have many similarities. Imagery allows you to pray in whatever way is right for you.
+ A contemplation of what came before life and what may come afterward can relieve a lot of fear around issues of mortality.
+ A guided imagery process will allow you to get a different perspective on these issues.

12

Cancer Free

Most people eagerly look forward to the end of treatment.
They expect to feel relieved and excited that treatment is over;
however, their reactions when treatment ends are often
surprising and different from what they expected.
—*Ernest Rosenbaum, M.D.*

The recovered patient is "weller than well."
—*O. Carl Simonton, M.D.*, The Healing Journey

The immediate post-treatment period is one that is often ignored in the care of many cancer patients. After weeks, months, or even years of close, caring attention from your doctors, your healers, and your support people, you are now pronounced in remission or cured, and it is almost as if everyone expects you to go back to normal, to how you were before you were ever diagnosed with cancer.

There's only one problem with this—you may or may not be the same as you were before. Some people, the "bump-in-the-roaders," move through the cancer experience without any seeming change in their personalities or philosophies, just as some men come home from war and pick up their lives where they left off. Most people, however, do not come back unchanged. What they have experienced forever alters their orientation to life, to themselves, and to others. Some are crushed and lapse into depression, anxiety, or common home remedies, such as drinking and drugs. Others learn they are capable of much more than they ever thought they were, that they can summon courage when they are afraid and are tougher than they believed.

Cancer survivors are similar to war veterans. Some feel that they have been through the biggest challenge that life can bring, and they get lazy and concentrate on taking it easy, waiting for their time to come, while others feel they have survived for a reason and rededicate their lives to what's important to them. Some bemoan the loss of the unusual closeness and camaraderie that occurs in times of war and times of cancer crisis, while others work hard to maintain the connections they developed during this time. Many never felt so loved, so cared for, and so reliant on others for their well-being as they have through this experience, and are surprised that there is an adjustment to returning to a life of greater safety but less intensity.

Rachel Naomi Remen, herself a survivor of a chronic illness, says that though an acute illness is stressful, it usually does not precipitate an identity shift, while a chronic illness, which most cancer is, often demands one. After the shock, numbness, denial, and anger you may have come to accept that you were a person with cancer, or a cancer patient. You took up that role and played it to the hilt, seeking the best care, multiple opinions, braving treatments and side effects, tolerating uncertainty, waiting, using all your resources and committing yourself fully to the fight. Now your treatment is over. Who are you now? Are you still a person with cancer? A person who *had* cancer? How do you define yourself now?

The emotional recovery from cancer can take longer than the physical recovery, and it may not even start until after the physical recovery. The person who has fought cancer has had an experience outside the normal sphere of life, like the soldier who has gone to war or the victim of an assault. It's called trauma. Even though two million Americans a year are diagnosed with some form of cancer, and there are more than twenty million Americans living who have or have had cancer, it is still an experience that the majority of people have not had. Trauma can remove the feeling of invincibility that we often take for granted and can make us aware of our vulnerability. For years afterward we can be more vigilant than we ever were, more anxious, more worried that an ache, pain, or bout of indigestion means the disease has recurred.

A survivor can feel betrayed and untrusting of his or her body and of life, yet it is equally possible at this stage to feel profound gratitude and awe for the ability of the body to withstand treatments, to tolerate discomfort, and to heal once again. Along with the experience of vulnerability can also come an appreciation of the courage and the ability to persevere and survive a life threat—a robustness that can increase your confidence in yourself and your connection to life.

It's all there—can you embrace it all? And which will you choose to energize?

You are a survivor, and your cancer is gone. Congratulations! Now you can start rebuilding your life. And if there is one good thing about cancer it is that it often offers you the opportunity to rebuild your life in a way that is better than it was before. If there are things you have always wanted to do but never did, this may be the time to pursue them (what other time is there?). If your priorities have changed during your cancer experience, then this is your chance to live with those reordered priorities; if they have not, it is your chance to once again pick up your work, your usual relationships, and daily activities.

Having had cancer, you may not be able to leave it behind for quite a while. You will probably be closely monitored to make sure any recurrence is picked up early. You may be seeing your oncologist every month, then every three months, then six months for several years. The exposure to the doctors, hospital, laboratory, X rays or MRI imaging may bring back memories and feelings of what it was like to go through your diagnosis and treatment. Using the mental tools you have developed will help you with this.

So now that your treatment is over, are you someone with cancer, or someone who has had cancer? Are you the same or different than you used to be? Do you want to be the same or different than you used to be?

In an unexpected way, you may find that you are again thrust into a new world of unknowing and find yourself again disoriented, a stranger in a strange land, much like the state you were in when you were first diagnosed. As you did before, acknowledge that this is a new phase and give yourself some time to explore it and find your way around. This too is a time when support can be important. If you don't have close friends or family to talk to, you may want to continue in a support group, especially if you can find one (or start one) for survivors. Alternatively, a pastoral counselor, psychotherapist, or physician familiar with these issues can be helpful. And it's a time when your imagery can be of great help, a time when your inner support can be invaluable.

The same skills you learned to use in fighting the cancer can now help you redefine, rebuild, and renew yourself. Your healing place is still a place of beauty, comfort, strength, and of healing. You may find that your healing place changes at this stage, or that you want to begin this new stage of life with a new place that brings you the energy and qualities you most cherish now. Trust your instincts about what feels most healthy for you now. You don't need to have an illness to welcome healing because every day we encounter challenges, we expend energy, we may even be wounded in our feelings if not our body. We spend our lives doing what we do, and coming to a healing place on a daily basis to draw from its healing energy can refresh and renew you even if you are in radiant good health.

If your Inner Healer was helpful to you in your fight, it can be even more helpful now in living a wise and loving life. You may continue with the Inner Healer that helped you this far, or find a new inner guide to walk with in the next part of the life path.

If your healing place or Inner Healer changes at this juncture, make sure to thank both your old healing place and Inner Healer for what they have brought you. Express the appreciation you have for them and ask if you can call on them again if you need them. If you feel you want to stay with these images, then ask your Inner Healer what would be most helpful to you now.

If you find that you worry a great deal about having a recurrence, use the Worry Warrior script from chapter 2. Remember, if a symptom or worry develops that doesn't go away in a week, get it thoroughly checked out by your doctor, but otherwise notice your fear and evoke instead the image you have (or will form shortly) of your healthiest self, the self you envision to be ideal. This way you can turn your worries to intentions, your fears to actions.

Depending on what type and stage of cancer you had, you may be physically unchanged or you may have lost some part of your physical body or its function and will need to integrate that into your new life. If you have gone through cytotoxic treatments, it may take a while to build your strength and resilience. It's not unusual for this to take a year or more, though in many cases, with good nutrition, rest when you are tired, and appropriate movement and exercise, it takes less time than that. Use Evocative Imagery, which you learned in chapter 3, to build strengths and qualities that will help you make real your ideal healthy self, and continue to write goals for yourself. You may want to start a new journal, perhaps a Healthy Living Journal, or a Happy Living Journal, or whatever you would like to call it. Remember the strengths and skills you've found and cultivated in yourself during this struggle—they can remain lifelong friends and help you create the life you'd like for yourself.

The following imagery process will give you a chance to revisit your healing place, your Inner Healer, and any other inner support that has sustained you through your treatment. It will invite you to let images arise of yourself before cancer, yourself now, and yourself as you would ideally like to be in the future. It will give you a chance to get your bearings in this journey and set your sights on where you want to go now that you are free of cancer.

Living Healthy and Well

Take a comfortable position and let yourself begin to relax in your own way . . . let your breathing get a little deeper and fuller . . . but still comfortable . . . with every breath in, notice that you bring in fresh air, fresh oxygen, fresh energy that fuels your body . . . and with every breath out, imagine that you can release a bit of tension . . . a bit of discomfort . . . a bit of worry . . . and let that deeper breathing and the thoughts you have of fresh energy in and tension and worry out be an invitation to your body and mind to begin to relax . . . to begin to shift gears . . . and let it be an easy and natural movement . . . without having to force anything . . . without having to make anything happen right now . . . just letting it happen . . . just breathing and relaxing . . . breathing and energizing. . . .

Come back to taking a few deeper breaths whenever you feel like relaxing even more deeply . . . but for now, let your breathing take its own natural rate and its own natural rhythm . . . and simply let the gentle movement of your body as it breathes allow you to relax naturally and comfortably . . . almost without having to try. . . .

And noticing how your right foot feels right now . . . and how your left foot feels . . . and noticing that just before you probably weren't aware of your feet at all . . . but now that you turn your attention to them, you can notice them and how they feel . . . and notice the intelligence that is there in your feet . . . and notice what happens when you silently invite your feet to relax . . . and become soft and at ease . . . and in the same way noticing the intelligence in your legs and releasing your legs . . . and letting the intelligence in your legs respond in their own way . . . and noticing any release and relaxation that happens . . . without having to make any effort at all . . . just softening and releasing . . . and letting it be a comfortable and very pleasant experience. . . .

And you can relax even more deeply and comfortably if you want to . . . by continuing to notice the intelligence in different parts of your body and inviting them to soften and relax . . . and noticing how they relax . . . and you are in control of your relaxation and only relax as deeply as is comfortable for you . . . and if you ever need to return your awareness to the outer world you can do that by opening your eyes and looking around and coming fully alert . . . and if you need to respond to anything there you can do that . . . and knowing that you can do this if you need to . . . you can relax again and return your attention to the inner world of your imagination. . . .

Inviting the intelligence of your low back, pelvis, and hips to release and relax . . . and your abdomen and midsection . . . and your chest and rib cage . . . without effort or struggle . . . just letting go but staying aware as you do. . . .

Inviting the intelligence in your back and spine to soften and release . . . in your low back . . . mid-back . . . between and across your shoulder blades . . . and across your neck and shoulders . . . the intelligence in your arms . . . and elbows . . . and forearms . . . through your wrists and hands . . . and the palms of the hands . . . the fingers . . . and thumbs. . . .

Noticing the intelligence in your face and jaws and inviting them to relax . . . to become soft and at ease . . . and your scalp and forehead . . . and your eyes . . . even your tongue can be at ease. . . .

And as you relax, let your attention shift from your usual outer world to what we can call your inner world . . . the world inside that only you can see, hear, smell, and feel . . . the world where your memories, your dreams, your feelings, your plans all reside . . . a world that you can learn to connect with . . . that can help you in many ways on your journey. . . .

And imagine that you find inside a very special place . . . a very beautiful place where you feel comfortable and relaxed, yet very aware . . . this may be a place that you have actually visited at some time in your life . . . in the outer world or even in this inner world . . . or it may be a place that you've seen somewhere . . . or it may be a brand-new place that you haven't visited before . . .

and none of that matters as long as it is a very beautiful place, a place that invites you and feels good to be in . . . a place that feels safe and healing for you. . . .

And let yourself take some time to explore this place . . . and notice what you imagine seeing there . . . all the things you see . . . and how you see them . . . don't worry at all about how you imagine this place as long as it is beautiful to you and feels safe and healing . . . and notice if there are any sounds you imagine hearing . . . or if it is simply very quiet in your healing place . . . notice if there is a fragrance or aroma that you imagine there or a special quality of the air . . . there may or may not be, and it's perfectly all right however you imagine this place of healing . . . it may change over time as you explore it, or it may stay the same . . . it doesn't matter at this point . . . just let yourself explore a little more. . . .

Can you tell what time of day it is? . . . or what time of year it is? . . . and what the temperature is like? . . . how you are dressed? . . . take some time to find a place where you feel safe and let yourself get comfortable there . . . and just notice how it feels to imagine yourself there . . . and if your mind wanders from time to time, just take another deep breath or two and gently return your attention to this beautiful and healing place . . . just for now . . . without feeling the need to go anywhere else right now . . . or do anything else . . . just for now. . . .

And allow yourself to become aware of anything here that feels healing to you . . . it may be the beauty . . . it may be the sense of peacefulness . . . it may be the temperature, or the fragrance, or a combination of all the qualities that are here . . . perhaps you have a sense of what's sacred to you and what supports you in your life . . . it doesn't matter what you find healing here . . . or whether you can even identify it specifically . . . but let yourself experience whatever healing is there for you . . . and simply relax there . . . and know that while you relax, your body's natural healing and defense systems can operate at their highest efficiency . . . without distraction . . . and without needing to be told what to do. . . .

As you are enjoying this comfortable state of relaxation and healing, invite an image for any inner support you have to be with you . . . an Inner Healer . . . or images of people that are genuinely supportive of your healing . . . or of whatever spiritual force supports and guides you . . . and ask for their help in beginning to imagine yourself as you were before cancer, as you are now, and as you would ideally like to be in the near future. . . .

First, allow an image to come to mind that represents how you were before your cancer diagnosis . . . this may look like you or may be a symbol that represents something important to notice about the way you were . . . and take some time to observe this image . . . what does it look like? . . . how is its vitality? . . . what stands out to you? . . . is there any clue that this person might be vulnerable to cancer as it looks now? . . . what do you notice that might indicate a vulnerability? . . . what do you notice about this image that you value? . . . how do you feel toward this image? . . . and what are your thoughts about it? . . . is there anything you'd like it to know? . . . if so, express that directly to it . . . and let it respond to you . . . what does it want you to know? . . . what does it have in it that you dearly love and want to maintain? . . . and is there anything it embodies that you'd like to leave behind? . . .

Now allow another image to emerge that represents you now . . . again, this may be an image of you or some symbol that can communicate something important for you to know . . . remember, this is simply you now . . . at one point in a process of change and development . . . so let it be what it is . . . and take some time to observe it carefully. . . .

What does it look like? . . . how is its vitality? . . . what stands out to you? . . . what do you notice about it that's different than the other image? . . . what do you notice about this image that you value? . . . how do you feel toward this image? . . . and what are your thoughts about it? . . . is there anything you'd like it to know? . . . if so, express that directly to it . . . and let it respond to you . . . what does it want you to know? . . . what does it have in it that you dearly love and want to maintain? . . . and is there anything it embodies that you'd like to leave behind? . . .

And now allow yourself to imagine yourself completely well . . . with all the energy you can imagine yourself having . . . expressing the qualities you most value in every gesture, comment, and action . . . notice what this is like for you . . . notice the physical appearance of this radiantly healthy you . . . and how you are dressed . . . imagine yourself dressed as you would most like to dress . . . in clothes that genuinely express your nature and feel good to be in . . . notice how you move and what you see in your eyes and face as you manifest this excellent health and vitality . . . let this image be one of substance . . . an image of good health deep down and all the way through . . . imagining that the healthy vitality and qualities you value penetrate deep down into the very marrow . . . the bones . . . the muscles and ligaments . . . the organs within your pelvis . . . abdomen . . . chest . . . through your face and skull . . . your brain . . . spinal cord and nerves . . . your blood cells and immune cells . . . and all the way out to the outermost layers of your skin . . . if it feels good to you, imagine that this energy permeates the space around you for several feet in every direction . . . whatever distance seems ideal to you . . . the ideal balance between projecting and absorbing. . . .

Notice how this healthiest self interacts with others . . . those that are easy to interact with . . . and those that are more difficult . . . and imagine that it can say yes or no with equal skill . . . and that it can somehow easily balance the needs of others with its own needs . . . and be graceful yet firm in doing this . . . and imagine what it would be to live in a way that balanced energy expended with energy absorbed . . . and who would have to be involved in conversations to make this happen . . . and how that could be done successfully. . . .

You might imagine moving into this image and becoming it for a while . . . notice what you feel in your body as you try on this healthy image . . . as you might an outfit . . . trying it on for size and fit . . . and feel free to adjust it and add anything to it that feels even better . . . and notice whether it fits you now or there is some growing into it that needs to happen . . . either way is fine. . . .

And if it fits you now, let yourself remember to access this image to affirm the healthy you now . . . and if there is some healing and strengthening yet to do, imagine how you will support that so you can enjoy this optimum health fully and soon. . . .

And notice how it feels to affirm that you are free of cancer . . . and building health and vitality . . . and that you can come out of this experience stronger and healthier than you were when you entered it . . . and that you have learned ways to strengthen the healing and defense abilities of your body now and they can stay alert and aware and eliminate any threat to your good health in the future. . . .

And that you are more aware now than ever of the preciousness and value of life . . . and it fuels every day with a curiosity, a joy and gratefulness that you may not have had before . . . and makes every day a day to live fully . . . and enjoyable . . . and with all the love and wisdom you can access. . . .

Taking all the time you need. . . .

And when you are ready to return your attention to the outer world, silently express any appreciation you might have for having a special healing place within you . . . and for being able to use your imagination in this way . . . and for the healing capabilities that have been built into you by nature . . . and for the treatments that have helped you eliminate cancer . . . and when you are ready, allow all the images to fade and go back within . . . knowing that healing continues to happen within you at all times . . . and gently bring your attention back to the room around you and the current time and place . . . and bring back with you anything that seems important or interesting to bring back, including any feelings of comfort, relaxation, or healing . . . and when you are all the way back, gently stretch and open your eyes. . . .

And take a few minutes to write or draw about your experience.

Debriefing Your Experience

As usual, write or draw what seemed significant or interesting to you about this experience. Following that, answer the following, if you haven't already:

How do you feel after doing this process?

How did you imagine yourself before cancer?

What did you notice or learn about yourself then from this imagery?

What qualities did you have then that you value?

What, if any, did you want to leave behind?

How did you imagine yourself now?

What did you notice or learn about yourself now from this imagery?

What qualities do you have that you value?

What, if any, do you want to leave behind?

How did you imagine your ideally healthy self?

What qualities does it have that you value?

How did it feel to be this ideal self?

How close or far away to feeling like this do you seem?

What can you do in your daily life to bring yourself closer to actually being this way?

What seemed most important or interesting to you about your imagery this time?

What do you know about yourself now that you didn't before?

What above all do you want to remember from this cancer experience?

What especially did you learn that could keep you healthy in the future?

When you take on your cancer with a willing spirit and come through cancer-free, you often end up healthier, stronger, happier, and more philosophical than you were before, even though regaining your physical strength and endurance may take some time. Set your sights now on good health and happiness, unless there is something more important to you, and then set your sights on those things. Practice what helped you to survive and you can take your well-being to levels you may not have previously ever dreamed.

Summary

- The period after treatment is over presents its own challenges even when you are free of cancer.
- The same skills you learned to help you fight cancer can help you rebuild your life and vitality, and come out of this experience stronger and wiser than you were before.
- Cancer may offer an opportunity for you to make your life the way you want it to be.

Notes

Introduction

1. Richardson, M. A., Post-White, J., Grimm, E. A., Moye, L. A., Singletary, S. E., and Justice B. Coping, life attitudes, and immune responses to imagery and group support after breast cancer treatment. *Alternative Therapies in Health and Medicine* 3(5) (1997): 62–70.

2. Gruber, B. L., Hersh, S. P., Hall, N. R., Waletzky, L. R., Kunz, J. F., Carpenter, J. K., Kverno, K. S., and Weiss, S. M. Immunological responses of breast cancer patients to behavioral interventions. *Biofeedback and Self Regulation*, 18(1) (March 1993): 1–22; Hall, H., Minnes, L., and Olness, K. The psychophysiology of voluntary immunomodulation. *International Journal of Neuroscience* 69(1–4) (March–April 1993): 221–34.

3. Tusek, D. L. Guided Imagery; a significant advance in the care of patients undergoing elective colorectal surgery. *Diseases of the Colon and Rectum*, 40(2) (1997): 172–78; Disbrow, E. A., Bennett, H. L., and Owings, J. T. Preoperative suggestion hastens the return of gastrointestinal mobility. *Western Journal of Medicine* 158 (5) (May 1993): 488–92.

4. Syrjala, K. L., et al. Relaxation and imagery and cognitive-behavioral training reduce pain during cancer treatment: a controlled clinical trial. *Pain* 63 (1995): 189–98; Integration of behavioral and relaxation approaches into the treatment of chronic pain and insomnia. NIH Technology Assessment Panel on Integration of Behavioral and Relaxation Approaches into the Treatment of Chronic Pain and Insomnia. *JAMA* (*Journal of the American Medical Association*) 276(4) (July 24–31, 1996): 313–18.

5. Troesch, L. M., et al. The influence of guided imagery on chemotherapy-related nausea and vomiting. *Oncology Nursing Forum* 20(8) (September, 1993): 1179–85; Burish, T. G., Conditioned side effects induced by cancer chemotherapy: Prevention through behavioral treatment. *J Consulting & Clinical Psychology* 55(1) (February 1987): 42–48.

1: Cancer Diagnosis: Nightmare, Challenge, or Bump in the Road?

1. Watson, M., Haviland, J. S., Greer, S., Davidson, J., Bliss, J. M. Influence of psychological response on survival in breast cancer: a population-based cohort study. *Lancet* 354(9187) (1999):1331–36.

2. Cassileth, B. R., Walsh, W. P., and Lusk, E. J. Psychosocial correlates of cancer survival: a subsequent report 3 to 8 years after cancer diagnosis. *J Clin Oncol* 6(11) (1988): 1753–59.

3. Randomization and matching are two methods for eliminating bias in a study. When patients are randomly selected to be either in the treatment group or control (no treatment) group, it eliminates the effect of people choosing what they think will work best for them. When patients in each group are "matched" to each other for age, gender, and stage of disease, that makes it more likely that any survival differences are due to the intervention.

4. Fawzy, F. I., Fawzy, N. W., Hyun, C. S., Elashoff, R., Guthrie, D., Fahey, J. L., and Morton, D. L. Malignant melanoma. Effects of an early structured psychiatric intervention, coping, and affective state on recurrence and survival 6 years later. *Arch Gen Psychiatry* 50(9) (September 1993): 681–89.

5. Shrock, D., Palmer, R. F., and Taylor, B. Effects of a psychosocial intervention on survival among patients with stage I breast and prostate cancer: a matched case-control study. *Alternative Therapies in Health and Medicine* 5(3) (1999): 49–55.

6. Cunningham, A. J., Edmonds, C. V., Phillips, C., Soots, K. I., Hedley, D., and Lockwood, G. A. A prospective, longitudinal study of the relationship of psychological work to duration of survival in patients with metastatic cancer. *Psychooncology* 9(4): 323–39.

2: After Diagnosis: The First Three Weeks

1. Newell, S., et al. How well do medical oncologists' perceptions reflect their patients' reported physical and psychosocial problems? Data from a survey of five oncologists. *Cancer* 83(8) (1998): 1640–51.

3: Combating the Stress of Cancer

1. "Complementary" refers to treatments that support your health and complement your treatment, "alternative" refers to treatments chosen instead of conventional treatment.

2. Rosenbaum, Ernest H., M.D., and Rosenbaum, Isadora R., M.A. *Supportive Cancer Care: The Complete Guide for Patients and Their Families.* Sourcebooks Trade, 2001.

3. Classen, C., Butler, L. D., Koopman, C., Miller, E., DiMiceli, S., Giese-Davis, J., Fobair, P., Carlson, R. W., Kraemer, H. C., and Spiegel, D. Supportive-expressive group therapy and distress in patients with metastatic breast cancer: a randomized clinical intervention trial. *Arch Gen Psychiatry* 58(5) (2001): 494–501.

4. Benson, H., and Wallace, R. The physiology of meditation. *Scientific American* 226 (1972): 84–90.

5. http://www.cdc.gov/ncbddd/bd/faq1.htm

4: Why Is Imagery Important?

1. Hall, H., Minnes, L., and Olness, K. The psychophysiology of voluntary immunomodulation. *International Journal of Neuroscience* 69(1–4) (March–April 1993): 221–34.

2. Frank, J. *Persuasion and Healing*. New York: Schocken Books, 1974.

3. Levine, J. D., Gordon, N. C., and Fields, H. L. The mechanism of placebo analgesia. *Lancet* 2(8091) (September 1978): 654–57.

4. Achterberg, J. *Imagery in Healing*. Boston: New Science Library, Shambala, 1985.

5. Nucho, A. *Spontaneous Creative Imagery: Problem-Solving and Life-Enhancing Skills*. Springfield, Ill.: Charles C. Thomas, 1995.

6. Chang, E., translator. *Knocking at the Gate of Life and Other Healing Exercises from China: The Official Handbook of the People's Republic of China*. Emmaus, Pa.: Rodale Press, 1985.

7. Donden, Y. *Health through Balance: An Introduction to Tibetan Medicine*. Ithaca, N.Y.: Snow Lion Publications, 1986.

8. Scholem, G. *Major Trends in Jewish Mysticism*. New York: Schocken Books, 1961.

9. Pert, C. B. *Molecules of Emotion: Why You Feel the Way You Feel*. New York: Scribner, 1997.

10. McMahon, C., and Sheikh, A. Imagination in disease and healing processes: a historical perspective, in *Imagination and Healing*, Sheikh, A., ed. Farmingdale, N.Y.: Baywood Publishing, 1984.

11. McMahon, C., Halstrup, J. L. The role of imagination in the disease process: post-Cartesian history. *Journal of Behavioral Medicine* 36(2) (June 1980): 205–17.

12. Meissner, W. W., Mack, J. E., and Semrad, E. V., in *Comprehensive Textbook of Psychiatry II*, vol. I, 2nd ed., Freedman, A. M., Kaplan, H. I., and Sadock, B. J., eds. Baltimore, Md.: Williams & Wilkins, 1975.

13. Ibid.

14. Jung, C. G. *The Practice of Psychotherapy*, Bollingen Series XX. Princeton, N.J.: Princeton University Press, 1966, p. 11.

15. Assagioli, R. *Psychosynthesis*. New York: The Viking Press, 1965, pp. 11–21.

16. Holt, R. R. Imagery: the return of the ostracized. *American Psychologist* 19 (1964): 254–64.

5: *Stimulating Healing*

1. Smyth, J. M., Stone, A. A., Hurewitz, A., and Kaell, A. Effects of writing about stressful experiences on symptom reduction in patients with asthma or rheumatoid arthritis: a randomized trial. *JAMA* 281(14) (April 1999): 1304–09.

2. Gaynor, M. *The Healing Power of Sound: Recovery from Life-Threatening Illness Using Sound, Voice and Music.* Boston: Shambala Publications, 2002.

7: *Preparing for Successful Surgery*

1. Blue Shield report to National Managed Health Care Congress, Baltimore, Md., 2002.

2. Disbrow, E. A., Bennett, H. L., and Owings, J. T. Preoperative suggestion hastens the return of gastrointestinal mobility. *Western Journal of Medicine* 158(5) (May 1993): 488–92.

3. Bennett, H. L., Benson, D. R., and Kuiken, D. A. Preoperative instructions for decreased bleeding during spine surgery. *Anesthesiology* 65 (1986): A245.

8: *Making the Most of Chemotherapy*

1. Giang, D. W., Goodman, A. D., Schiffer, R. B., Mattson, D. H., Petrie, M., Cohen, N., and Ader, R. Conditioning of cyclophosphamide-induced leukopenia in humans. *J Neuropsychiatry Clin Neurosci* 8(2) (Spring 1996): 194–201.

2. Morrow, G. R., and Morrell, C. Behavioral treatment for the anticipatory nausea and vomiting induced by cancer chemotherapy. *NEJM* (*New England Journal of Medicine*) 307 (1982): 1476–80.

3. Marchioro, G., Azzarello, G., Viviani, F., Barbato, F., Pavanetto, M., Rosetti, F., Pappagallo, G. L., and Vinante O. Hypnosis in the treatment of anticipatory nausea and vomiting in patients receiving cancer chemotherapy. *Oncology* 59(2) (August 2000): 100–104; Jacknow, D. S., Tschann, J. M., Link, M. P., and Boyce, W. T. Hypnosis in the prevention of chemotherapy-related nausea and vomiting in children: a prospective study. *J Dev Behav Pediatr* 15(4) (August 1994): 258–64.

4. Syrjala, K. L., Donaldson, G. W., Davis, M. W., Kippes, M. E., and Carr, J. E. Relaxation and imagery and cognitive-behavioral training reduce pain during cancer treatment: a controlled clinical trial. *Pain* 63(2) (November 1995): 189–98.

5. Walker, L. G., Walker, M. B., Ogston, K., Heys, S. D., Ah-See, A. K., Miller, I. D., Hutcheon, A. W., Sarkar, T. K., and Eremin O. Psychological, clinical and pathological effects of relaxation training and guided imagery during primary chemotherapy. *British Journal of Cancer* 80(1–2) (April 1999): 262–68.

6. Newell, S., et al. How well do medical oncologists' perceptions reflect their patients' reported physical and psychosocial problems? Data from a survey of five oncologists. *Cancer* 83(8) (1998): 1640–51.

7. Syrjala, K. L., Donaldson, G. W., Davis, M. W., Kippes, M. E., and Carr, J. E. Op cit.

9: Making the Most of Radiation Therapy and Other Treatments

1. Kolcaba, K., Fox C. The effects of guided imagery on comfort of women with early stage breast cancer undergoing radiation therapy. *Oncology Nursing Forum* 26(1) (January–February 1999): 67–72.

2. Walker, L. G., Walker, M. B., Ogston, K., Heys, S. D., Ah-See, A. K., Miller, I. D., Hutcheon, A W., Sarkar, T. K., and Eremin, O. Psychological, clinical and pathological effects of relaxation training and guided imagery during primary chemotherapy. *British Journal of Cancer* 80(1–2) (April 1999): 262–68.

10: Relieving Pain

1. Syrjala, K. L., et al. Relaxation and imagery and cognitive-behavioral training reduce pain during cancer treatment: a controlled clinical trial. *Pain* 63 (1995): 189–98; Sloman, R. The use of relaxation for the promotion of comfort and pain relief in persons with advanced cancer. *Contemporary Nurse* 3(1) (1994): 6–12; Sloman, R. Relaxation and the relief of cancer pain. *Nursing Clinics of North America* 30(4) (1995): 697–709; Breitbart, W. Psychiatric management of cancer pain. *Cancer* 63(11 suppl) (June 1, 1989): 2336–42; Daake, D. R. Imagery instruction and the control of postsurgical pain. *Applied Nursing Research* 2(3) (August 1989): 114–20; Frank, J. *Persuasion and Healing*. New York: Schocken Books, 1974.

11: Spiritual Aspects of Cancer and Healing

1. Sicher, F., Targ, E., Moore, D., II, and Smith, H. S. A randomized double-blind study of the effect of distant healing in a population with advanced AIDS. Report of a small scale study. *Western Journal of Medicine* 169(6) (December 1998): 356–63.

2. Byrd, R. C. Positive therapeutic effects of intercessory prayer in a coronary care unit population. *Southern Medical Journal* 159(7) (July 1988): 826–29.

3. Harris, W. S., Gowda, M., Kolb, J. W., Strychacz, C. P., Vacek, J. L., Jones, P. G., Forker, A., O'Keefe, J. H., and McCallister, B. D. A randomized, controlled trial of the effects of remote, intercessory prayer on outcomes in patients admitted to the coronary care unit. *Archives of Internal Medicine* 159(19) (October 25, 1999): 2273–78.

4. Sicher, F., Targ, E., Moore, D. II, and Smith, H. S. A randomized double-blind study of the effect of distant healing in a population with advanced AIDS. Report of a small scale study. *Western Journal of Medicine* 169(6) (December 1998): 356–63.

Resources

Finding a Certified Interactive Guided Imagery[sm] *Guide*

The Academy for Guided Imagery
P.O. Box 2070
Mill Valley, CA 94942
800-726-2070
www.interactiveimagery.com

Audio and Video Recordings

Fighting Cancer from Within Audio Series
All fifteen guided imagery processes taught in this book are professionally recorded for you by Dr. Rossman. Available as a CD or a cassette set. Order through the Imagery Store at 800-726-2070 or www.interactiveimagery.com

Simonton Cancer Center
Tapes and Literature Department
P.O. Box 623
Bridgeport, TX 76426
800-338-2360
email: simonton@wf.net

Health Journeys
Tapes by Belleruth Naparstek
www.healthjourneys.com

Emmett Miller, M.D. tapes
www.drmiller.com

Bernie Siegel, M.D. tapes
www.peoplesuccess.com

Books

Getting Well Again, O. Carol Simonton, M.D., Stephanie Matthews, James L. Creighton, Bantam, May 1992
The classic book that launched the modern era of interest in imagery and mind-body influences in cancer.

The Complete Cancer Survival Guide: Everything You Must Know and Where to Go for State-of-the-Art Treatment of the 25 Most Common Forms of Cancer, Peter Teeley, Philip Bashe, Main Street Books, April 2000
This 972-page encyclopedic work is a useful reference describing current conventional approaches to treating cancer. It encourages mind-body work but doesn't teach it.

Comprehensive Cancer Care: Integrating Alternative, Complementary and Conventional Therapies, James Gordon, M.D., Sharon Curtin, Perseus, May 2000
Dr. Gordon has sponsored the groundbreaking Comprehensive Cancer Care conferences in Washington, D.C., bringing the best of conventional and complementary cancer care together under the auspices of the National Cancer Institute and M. D. Anderson Cancer Center. An excellent guide for navigating the process of integrating your care.

The Journey through Cancer: An Oncologist's Seven-Level Program for Healing and Transforming the Whole Person, Jeremy Geffen, M.D., Crown, February 2000
A beautifully written book by a leading integrative oncologist that stresses attending to mind, emotions, and spirit as crucial to whole person cancer care.

Complementary Cancer Therapies: Combining Traditional and Alternative Approaches for the Best Possible Outcome, Dan Labriola, Prima, January 2000
Another useful book that makes a strong case for integrating mind-body-spirit approaches into cancer care.

Rituals of Healing: Using Imagery for Health and Wellness, Jeanne Achterberg, Ph.D., Barbara Dossey, R.N., Leslie Kolkmeier, Bantam Doubleday Dell, May 1994

An excellent book teaching guided imagery rituals for a variety of common illnesses and conditions, including cancer. Supports the intelligent use of imagery for healing.

Cancer as a Turning Point: A Handbook for People with Cancer, Their Families, and Health Professionals, Lawrence LeShan, revised edition, Plume, December 1999
An inspiring book by the grandfather of psychological work with cancer patients that encourages them to find the things that turn them on and give them reasons to live.

Love, Medicine and Miracles, Bernie Siegel, M.D., Harper Perennial, June 1990
The classic inspirational book by the renowned cancer surgeon-healer. Has encouraged many people to accept their diagnosis, but not their prognosis.

Spontaneous Healing, Andrew Weil, M.D., Fawcett Columbine, May 1995
This book allowed us to think about the healing potential of the mind and body in a new way, and laid the ground for the rational inclusion of life-strengthening therapies and practices in the treatment of illness, including cancer.

Healing Words, Larry Dossey, M.D., Harper Collins, 1993
A scientific investigation of the ability of prayer to affect the healing process. Drawn from the extensive research and observations of a foremost authority on the interface between orthodox and alternative medicine.

Residential Programs

The Simonton Cancer Center
P.O. Box 890
Pacific Palisades, CA 90272
800-459-3424
info@simontoncenter.com

Cancer as a Turning Point Intensive Workshops (Larry LeShan, Ph.D.)
www.cancerasaturningpoint.org

The Commonweal Cancer Help Program
www.commonweal.org/cchp

Research Services

The Moss Reports
144 St. John's Place
Brooklyn, NY 11217
718-636-0186
http://www.ralphmoss.com

Ralph Moss, Ph.D., is a science writer and a vocal advocate of alternative approaches to cancer. His Moss Reports are custom reports personally researched, written, and updated by Dr. Moss for a wide range of cancer diagnoses. Each report features complementary and alternative treatments for your type of cancer, such as nutritional, immunological, herbal, and biological approaches; an overview of your conventional treatment options; an assessment of your chances for success with those treatments; information on which supplements you should avoid; and more. Resources are given, including the names, addresses, and phone numbers of practitioners who may be able to help.

CANHELP
www.canhelp.com

Patrick McGrady assists patients to make informed decisions regarding cancer treatments. McGrady has assembled a network of practitioners in the area of complementary treatment for cancer to provide you and/or your physicians with up-to-date data and an understanding of the range of treatment options that lie outside the mainstream. For a fee, patients can receive a CANHELP packet that contains a computer printout of relevant research and treatment information from medical databases, a personal interpretation of these data for you and your physician, and a synopsis of conversations on your behalf with CANHELP's network of medical advisors.

Internet Resources

American Cancer Society
www.cancer.org

This site features a bookstore, links to important cancer organizations, information about complementary and alternative treatments, and access to the Cancer Survivors Network, which allows cancer patients to share information and resources that have been helpful to them.

Cancer Information Service of National Cancer Institute
http://www.nci.nih.gov

This government site offers conventional cancer information and also links to the National Center for Complementary and Alternative Medicine site, which provides information about guided imagery.

Cancer Supportive Care Program
http://www.cancersupportivecare.com/psychosocial.html

This site is devoted to information for supporting the cancer patient and caregivers and emphasizes the roles of attitude, emotions, support groups, the power of the mind, nurturing hope, and improving coping skills. The information is even-handed and provided by such leaders in the field as David Spiegel, Ph.D., from Stanford, and Ernest Rosenbaum, M.D., from the University of California, San Francisco.

Cancer Survivor's Network
http://www.acscsn.org

A highly utilized site with support groups, chats, and shared information from and for cancer patients. Communication among cancer patients is an influential source of information and I have many grateful patients who have shared their experiences with imagery and cancer on this site.

National Coalition for Cancer Survivorship
1010 Wayne Avenue
Fifth Floor
Silver Spring, MD 20910
301-650-8868
http://www.cansearch.org

The National Coalition for Cancer Survivorship (NCCS) provides support for people wishing to locate or form self-help groups, assists survivors with insurance and employment problems, provides speakers on a wide range of topics, promotes the interests of survivors through the media, testifies in state and federal hearings, and provides a variety of publications of interest to survivors, including *The National Networking Directory of Cancer Support Services*. The NCCS also publishes the *Networker*, a quarterly newsletter that discusses issues affecting survivors.

Cancer Care, Inc.
1180 Avenue of the Americas
New York, NY 10036
212-302-2400 or 800–813-HOPE
http://www.cancercare.org/

Cancer Care is a nonprofit organization that provides a wealth of on-line, telephone, and referral services including medical referrals, second opinions, counseling, financial assistance information for non-medical expenses, and local support referrals, such as housekeeping and health aids. A free hotline offers immediate assistance with medical information, one-to-one counseling over the phone, referrals to services in your local area, and free educational materials. Services also include telephone access to educational programs and on-line support groups.

Self-Help Clearinghouse
Self-Help Sourcebook Online
http://www.mentalhelp.net/selfhelp

This comprehensive guide can act as a starting point for exploring support groups and networks that are available throughout the world for a whole array of health and other concerns, including cancer. The organizations listed in this directory can help you find and/or start a support group in your community. For a listing of online support groups and resources, select "cancer" in the Disorders and Treatment index available on the site.

Cancer Free Connections
http://www.cancer-free.com

A site with the stories of many well-known and not-so-well-known cancer survivors and their strategies and other resources available to people in the fight for life. The organization also publishes the newsletter *Options* and makes available a wide variety of educational materials, including books, articles, audio- and videotapes. Members and their companions may receive substantial discounts on medical travel costs.

CancerGuide: Alternative Therapies
http://cancerguide.org/alternative.html

This site written by cancer survivor Steve Dunn contains short evaluations of some of the better-known alternative cancer therapies that are available today and links to many complementary cancer centers. Dunn also provides information on how to search the medical literature, how to evaluate research, and how to decide if a clinical trial is right for you.

Ask Dr. Weil
http://cgi.pathfinder.com/@@ztzeJAQA@hWW8jiK/drweil/

Dr. Andrew Weil, the author of *Spontaneous Healing* and the director of the Integrative Medicine Program at the University of Arizona, gives well-balanced responses to questions from readers daily on his website.

Special thanks to Michael Lerner for his permission to use some of the website descriptions above from the Commonweal website, www.commonweal.org, a significant resource itself.

Acknowledgments

So many people's influences are woven into this book. There are the professionals who introduced me early in my career to the idea that imagery and the mind could influence the course of cancer: Carl Simonton, Stephanie Simonton-Matthews, Larry LeShan, Irving Oyle, Arthur Gladman, Ken Pelletier, Jeanne Achterberg, Karl Pribram, Jerome Frank, George Solomon, Norman Cousins, and David Bresler.

The researchers who have provided evidence that this is true: Fawzy Fawzy, David Spiegel, Alastair Cunningham, Dean Schrock, Elizabeth Targ, Howard Hall, and Karin Olness.

The patients too numerous to mention who have taught me so much about living with cancer, and healing from cancer, especially: Beyhan Lowman, Karinna Berner, Roy Mackenzie Sykes, Diane Brandon, Jerome Freedman, and David and Marilyn Weisberg.

My beloved family members who each fought battles with cancer: my father, Manny Rossman, my grandparents Lou and Jesse Shapero, my uncle Merrill Shapero, my uncle Harold Zuker, my aunt Rebecca Rabinowitz, my cousin Sheldon Rabinowitz, and my cousin Linda Coleman.

Colleagues who have advanced professional and public awareness of how the mind functions in healing: Andy Weil, Jim Gordon, Michael Lerner, Bernie Siegel, Deepak Chopra, Emmett Miller, Jimmie Holland, Jeremy Geffen, Jon Kabat-Zinn, Joan Borysenko, Larry Dossey, Barbara Dossey, Harris Dienstfrey, Sheldon Lewis, Bonnie Horrigan, Candace Pert, and Steven Locke.

Oncologists, physicians, and other health professionals who have long supported me with their active interest and encouragement in my work with people with cancer: Bill Fair, Keith Block, Dean Ornish, David Gullion, Peter Eisenberg, Debu Tripathy, Howard Rossman, Richard Shames, Elson Haas, Michael Broffman, Mark Renneker, Julia Rowland, and Christopher Sato-Perry.

Thanks to Keren Stronach and Diane Brandon for their feedback on the manuscript as well as their pioneering work supporting cancer patients, and special thanks to my assistant Ginny Stripp who makes my office life easy and helps me get what I need to get done.

My deepest appreciation goes to Rachel Naomi Remen, a spiritual warrior and friend of the finest sort, who took the precious time to write the foreword, as she has always taken time for me when needed.

Thanks to Arielle Eckstut, my agent, and Deborah Brody, my editor at Holt, for their belief in the value of this book.

Thanks above all to my family who support me and love me while I periodically turn my attention inward in order to write. Mie, Marisa, and Mariel, you know I love you more than words can say.

Index

Dr. Rossman's Fighting Cancer
From Within Guided Imagery CDs

Dr. Rossman is known for his soothing and inspiring voice as well as his work in guided imagery for healing. He has professionally recorded all the guided imagery processes in this book to make it easy for you to experiment and explore with them. Available as a complete set of CDs or audiotapes, these recordings will take you through each process, while you relax and let yourself become immersed in the process.

With express shipping these can be to you or your loved one in two days. Your satisfaction is guaranteed. If you don't feel these are helping you within thirty days, return them for a full refund.

Fighting Cancer from Within
5 CD set $69.95 x # units
Standard shipping & handling   7.00
Express shipping & handling   15.00
7.25% tax (California residents only)   5.07 x # units
Total

To order, send check or complete credit card information
(card type, name, number, exp. date) to:

FightCancerCDs
P.O. Box 1933
Mill Valley, CA 94942
Phone or fax: 1-415-389-8941
Email: FightCancerCDs@aol.com
www.fightcancerwithin.com

About the Author

Martin L. Rossman, M.D., is the cofounder and president of the Academy for Guided Imagery and is on the faculty of the medical school at the University California, San Francisco. The author of *Guided Imagery for Self-Healing*, he lives in Mill Valley, California.